AURAL CARE

Protocols and Guidelines

Third edition

Tristram Lesser MS FRCSEd
Consultant Otolaryngologist

Rebecca Donald
Advanced Nurse Practitioner

Aintree University Hospital Liverpool

ISBN-13:978-1502578099
ISBN-10:1502578093

Copyright © Tristram Lesser and Rebecca Donald 2016 All rights reserved

No part of this publication may be reproduced, stored in a retrieval system, or transmitted in any form or by any means, without the prior permission in writing of the publisher, nor be otherwise circulated in any form of binding or cover other than that in which it is published and without a similar condition including this condition being imposed on the subsequent purchaser.

AURAL CARE

Dedicated to all aural care practitioners and the ears they treat

ACKNOWLEDGMENTS

Thanks to Janet Robinson and Fiona Chew who contributed to the first and second editions of this book, Bob Duffy for his work on the previous editions, Paula Mitchell for her original art work on the cover and to Advanced Nurse Practitioners Lynn Robinson, Charlotte Halpin and Nicola Carmichael.

CONTENTS

1	Introduction	1
2	External Ear Conditions	6
3	Middle Ear Conditions	25
4	Inner ear Conditions	43
5	Otorrhoea	45
6	Before starting micro suction	49
7	Wax: Evidence Based Treatment	52
8	Guidelines	63
9	Protocols	84
10	Case Studies	89
11	References and Training Charts	95

1 INTRODUCTION

The third edition of Aural Care is produced at a time when nurse-led micro-suction aural care clinics have become the standard of care. Advanced Nurse Practitioners are now responsible for training aural care nurses and supervising them.

This guide describes the conditions treated, the criteria for training and the targets for the training of aural care nurses. It gives an example training program and advice on setting up and running a micro-suction clinic. As there is a need for integrated care between the primary care setting, where most wax removal is done, and secondary care, we provide the evidence-based guidelines for the management of wax.

The protocols are provided for aural micro-suction, removal of wax, treatment of otitis externa, care of mastoid cavities, furuncle treatment and removal of foreign body as well as administration of aural medications. It is important to remember that all such clinics need to be regularly audited. There are a few case studies to provide examples of prescribing for the ear and tables to be used for training.

NURSE-LED AURAL CARE

The UKCC published regulations in July 1992 which were designed to free the profession from the previous rules that limited nurses to basic, traditional duties. This new freedom led to the development of such roles as Nurse Practitioner and Clinical Nurse Specialists, roles requiring a high level of knowledge, expertise and practical ability in circumscribed, specialised areas. We now have many Advanced Nurse Practitioners in ENT who undertake the work previously done by doctors, treating emergencies, undertaking routine clinics and in some cases operating, as well as in the practice and supervision of aural care clinics

ENT out-patient nurses have taken advantage of the developments and opportunities available to expand their role and to complement the work of doctors in many areas. Nurse-led aural care is an important and exciting clinical development. Aural care has been performed in the past by nurses using direct vision and dry mopping techniques: micro-suction is, however, now the best available method of aural care for patients with many acute and chronic ear conditions.

Whilst nurses need to be accountable for their actions and only undertake care for which they feel adequately prepared, there are some formal, validated training courses in aural care. The development of the role should be under the direct supervision of the consultant in charge, who will ultimately take full responsibility for the treatments that the nurse gives. There are also basic issues that need to be considered before any training is undertaken:

- Education
- Accountability
- Support
- Motivation
- Assessment
- Maintenance of skills and the service

NURSE PRESCRIBING

An aural care clinic cannot function as nurse-led unless the nurse is able to provide the medications necessary to treat the patient. The issues surrounding nurse prescribing are many and protracted, but group protocols allow the nurse to supply and administer medications to patients who are not individually named but have the condition specified in the protocol.

A group protocol is a specific instruction for the supply and administration of a named medication in a named clinical situation. Protocols should be drawn up by a multidisciplinary team of doctors, pharmacists, nurses and managers.

Local requirements for protocols should be adhered to but there are basic requirements central to all:

- Description of the medication
- The clinical condition to which the protocol applies
- Detailed information on dosage, form, route, frequency and duration of administration
- Contra-indications and side effects
- Who can administer the medication
- Signatures of the doctor, pharmacist and manager
- Date the protocol was written and is due for review
- How records are to be kept and audited

ADVANCED NURSE PRACTITIONERS IN ENT

ENT advanced nurse practitioners will be expected undertake the modules in Nurse Prescribing and are able to prescribe outside specific protocols when undertaking supervision of aural care clinics or running them themselves. This would also include expectations to practise within a solid evidence base and to continually strive for service development.

2 EXTERNAL EAR CONDITIONS

EAR WAX

Epithelial migration

Body skin is constantly shed, usually as a result of friction from clothing or washing. To achieve this, skin grows continually from the depths to the surface and, as the dividing cells approach the outside, they die and shrink to become a waterproof layer. This surface layer is made waterproof by the presence of a protein called *keratin*. The dead surface layers of skin-cells are shed with wear and tear; on the scalp these scales of discarded skin are commonly known as dandruff.

This is not possible in the ear, as it would just fill with layers and layers of dead keratinised skin-cells. Consequently it has developed the special property of migration. All the skin starts growing at the centre of the tympanic membrane and migrates to the edges of the ear drum where it continues laterally. When it reaches the hair-bearing outer part of the canal the superficial layers separate. The skin then mixes with the secretion of the ceruminous and sebaceous glands to form ear wax. The glands are found in the skin of the outer third of the external acoustic meatus and secrete a liquid material at the base of the hairs. After secretion, evaporation occurs to leave a sticky, waxy substance that is able to trap dirt. Wax is protective since it kills many common and unpleasant bacteria and fungi, and generally stops insects and other foreign-bodies from inadvertently travelling down the ear canal.

Wax types and migration

Wax comes in one of two forms, wet and dry. Wet wax is moist, sticky and honey coloured, produced mainly by African and Caucasian ethnicities. This type of wax is genetically dominant. Dry wax is less genetically dominant and mainly produced by East Asian ethnicities. Its appearance is greyer and texture granular and flaky. Regardless of ethnicity ear wax tends to become naturally drier and harder with age. Wax is normally loosened by transmission of movement from the temporomandibular joint through chewing or talking, allowing its passage out of the ear. The migrating skin of the ear drum and ear canal moves laterally taking days to weeks to move skin and wax out. The "wax" that comes out is about 2/3rds skin and 1/3rd secretions. The natural process can be upset by a number of factors and cause wax impaction. Impaction is commoner in males owing to the presence of thicker, coarser hairs in the lateral part of the ear. Narrow canals, use of cotton buds and even a hearing aid mould may impede the normal flow of wax. Sometimes no obvious cause is found to account for the impaction.

Clinical features

Impaction of wax can cause a blocked feeling, deafness, pain, dizziness, itching, noises (tinnitus) and occasionally coughing (via the auricular branch of the vagus nerve, called *Arnold's nerve*). This nerve also explains why some people cough when their ear is cleaned. These symptoms can be improved by removing the wax.

Management

Uncomplicated wax impaction is usually treated within the primary care setting. A course of drops (sodium bicarbonate is effective, safe and inexpensive, sometimes olive oil but this is slightly less effective) is recommended prior to treatment. The wax is then expelled using a syringing technique, which involves a jet of body-temperature water being directed along the posterior superior (roof of) canal behind the wax and pushing it outwards.

Although relatively safe, complications such as coughing, pain, local trauma, otitis externa and rarely tympanic membrane perforation may occur.

There are contraindications to this type of removal: these conditions and their management are discussed following this section. Where these are present wax should only be removed using direct vision under a microscope with micro-suction and/or instrumentation, thus maximizing patient safety. This would usually be undertaken in, or linked to, a secondary care setting.

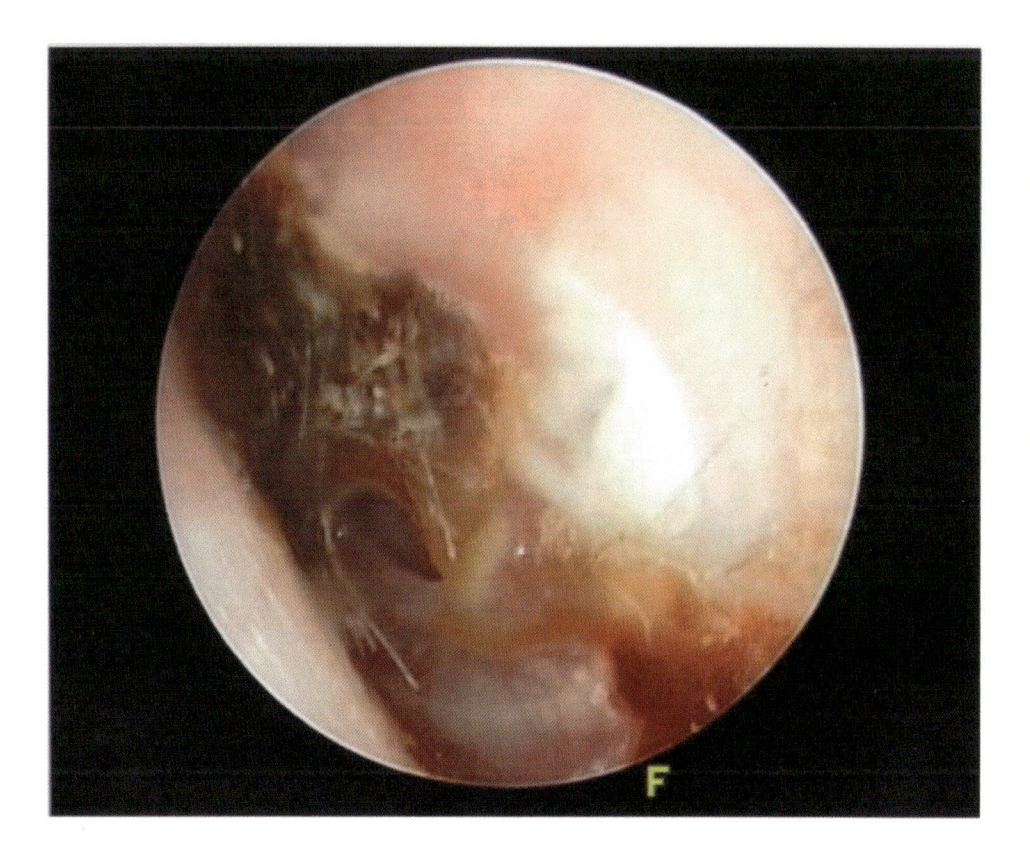

Left ear with wax and hairs pushed into the anterior recess and onto the drum by the patient cleaning the discharge from the small anterior perforation

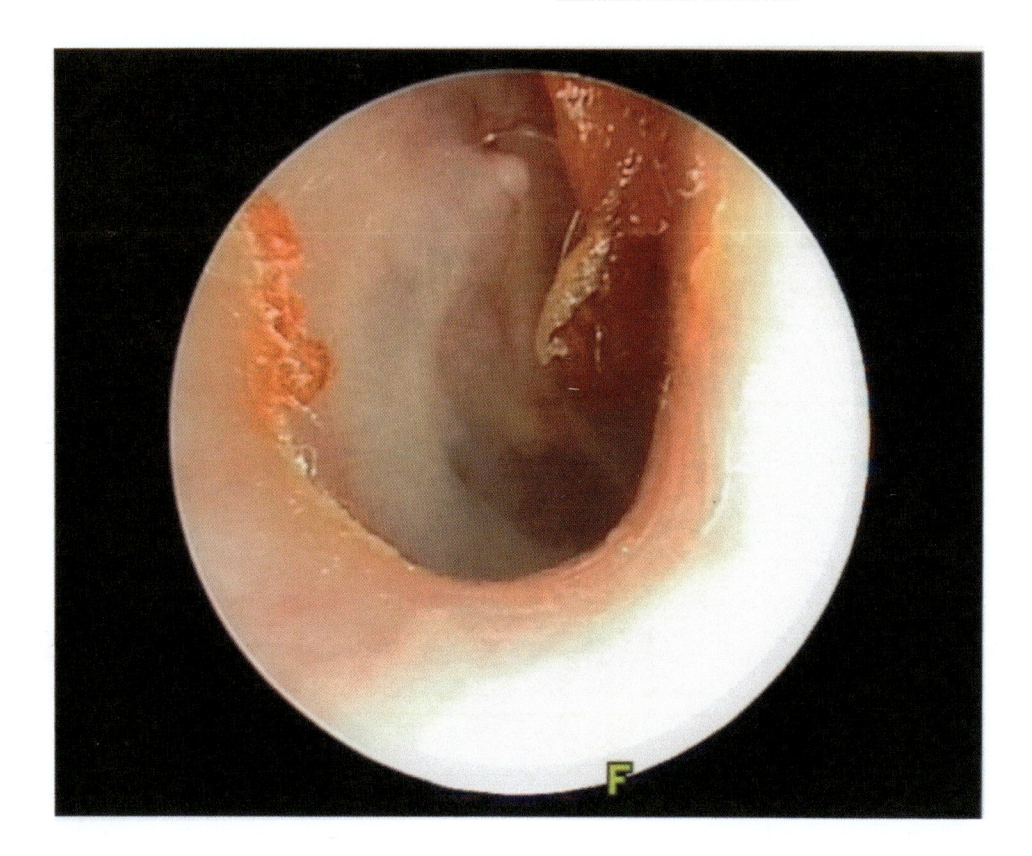

Wax in anterior recess; the ear drum is thickened by a previous myringoplasty

KERATOSIS OBTURANS

This uncommon condition occurs when there is a failure of the normal skin migration. Debris collects in the deep part of the external auditory meatus. As with collections of keratin anywhere, this sets up a low-grade inflammatory response resulting in a re-absorption of bone and widening of the bony canal.

Clinical Features

Patients usually present with an acute exacerbation of the inflammatory process. Pain is usually the dominant feature, although there is inevitably a hearing loss from the occluded canal. The appearance is similar to an acute otitis externa around impacted wax. The keratin takes this appearance because the part in contact with the air oxidizes and changes colour.

Management

Removal of the keratin plug is essential to control the inflammatory process. This is often difficult as the patient is usually in considerable pain and a general anaesthetic is often required. Topical antibiotic/steroid combinations are used to treat the secondary otitis externa. In the long term these patients require periodic aural toilet.

EXOSTOSES AND OSTEOMAS

Osteomas are uncommon benign round tumours of bone usually arising from the ear canal. Exostoses, on the other hand, are common. They are hyperostoses of the tympanic bone of the external canal and probably caused by a periosteal reaction to exposure to cold, usually from swimming. In both conditions, although the lumen of the canal is reduced, they rarely result in symptoms. If problems do occur they are usually related to impairment of the normal process of epithelial migration. In these cases surgical removal may be indicated. Osteomas can often be removed via the external canal, while exostoses will more often require a formal postaural or endaural approach. They are easy to diagnose as they are bony hard and hurt if prodded.

FOREIGN BODIES IN THE EAR

Foreign bodies are put into the ears more commonly by school children than by toddlers. The objects can be organic (pieces of paper, rubber, pencil, seeds, peas and beans) or inorganic (beads, buttons, crayons and stones). Inorganic foreign bodies are often asymptomatic, but organic objects may give rise to otitis externa by local irritation. One of the most common causes of this is cotton wool, and it is not unusual to find this in adult patients who have been attempting to clean their ears. Less common, but more irritating, are insects, either dead or dying.

Management

A foreign body in the external ear canal is usually seen on otoscopy. Removal may appear to be easy, but generally requires the skills and the facilities of a nurse specialist or ENT doctor. Ill-directed attempts atits removal by the untrained may lead to complications. It is usually possible to remove the foreign body in the clinic, but a general anaesthetic may be required for children and sensitive adults.

OTITIS EXTERNA

Otitis externa is defined as inflammation of the skin of the external auditory canal (EAC).

Acute otitis externa (AOE) is a condition consisting of infection and inflammation of the EAC. It is a common ENT problem, with a 12 month prevalence of over 1% in the UK and constituting one in six new patient referrals and 30% of follow-ups seen in one ENT emergency clinic. Infection is a major contributory factor to the condition, the commonest responsible organisms being Pseudomonas aeruginosa, Staphylococcus aureus and Staphylococcus epidermidis. It frequently occurs after the ear canal gets wet or following minor trauma to the ear canal. No national guidelines are currently available on the management of AOE.

The skin of the EAC has in its outer third an epithelial layer containing hair follicles, ceruminous glands and sebaceous glands, over a thin dermal layer containing sweat glands. This skin of the bony part of the canal lacks these and is very thin and tightly bound to the bone. The secretions of the sebaceous glands keep the skin watertight and supple.

Sweat gland secretions are acidic and keep the secretion at a pH between 3 and 5, which is lethal for most bacteria that are human pathogens. Usually the EAC contains Staphylococcus albus and other commensals, which can include pseudomonas organisms.

In the acute phase of otitis externa there are dilated skin blood vessels of increased permeability, which cause signs of a red, hot, oedematous and tender ear canal.

AURAL CARE

Predisposing factors:

- Heat, humidity, bathing, swimming

- Trauma, especially from dirty fingernails, cotton buds and hairgrips

- Inherited: narrow ear canals and certain blood types

- Dermatological conditions such as psoriasis, eczema and seborrhoeic dermatitis

- Loss of epithelial migration, loss of wax production

- Change in EAC pH

- Any combination of the above

Classification of Otitis Externa

1. Infective

    a)   Bacterial

    - Diffuse otitis externa commonly caused by Pseudomonas aeruginosa, Staphylococcus aureus and Proteus.

    - Furunculosis, usually caused by Staphylococcus aureus.

    - Necrotising otitis externa, usually caused by Pseudomonas aeruginosa or occasionally Staphylococcus aureusrysipelas caused by Streptococcus pyogenes.

    b)   Fungal

    - Aspergillus niger
    - Aspergillus fumigatus
    - Candida albicans

    c)   Viral

- Herpes simplex
- Herpes Zoster (Ramsey Hunt Syndrome)
- Presumptive in bullous haemorrhagica

2. Reactive

- Eczema
- Seborrhoeic dermatitis
- Allergy to drops
- Keratosis obturans
- Psoriasis
- Dandruff

Clinical Features

Otitis externa may be confined to the meatus (localized) or involve other areas of skin (generalized). Localised infection can be circumscribed or diffuse while generalized infection can be either primarily otological or primarily dermatological. There may be a history of direct trauma to the ear canal from swimming, ear 'cleaning' habits, atopic tendency and previous otological problems.

This history may provide a pointer towards the diagnosis:

- Severe itching suggests eczema, allergy or fungal infection;
- Pain occurs with furunculosis, diffuse otitis externa and herpes infections;
- Erythema is a feature of eczema, seborrhoeic dermatitis, or acute trauma;
- Vesicles occur in eczema and herpetic infection. Excess squamous debris suggests chronic eczema or fungal infection. Hypertrophic meatal skin suggests chronic disease.

It is not uncommon to find the ear canal closed by swelling in a patient with acute otalgia. A careful examination will usually distinguish furunculosis (common) from acute mastoiditis (now much less common). In the former there may be post-aural tenderness localized to a palpable lymph node. Exceptionally this node may break down to cause diffuse tenderness and oedema which may displace the pinna slightly forwards and invariably cause pain on moving the pinna. A patient with acute mastoiditis will have a more marked post-aural swelling, which may be fluctuant, displacing the pinna down as well as forwards. In this case there is less pain on moving the pinna and there will be a preceding history of acute suppurative otitis media.

Investigations

A culture swab should be taken for microbiological culture, including fungal culture, and antibiotic/antifungal sensitivity.

Management

In general practice topical antimicrobials, with or without topical steroids, should be the initial treatment of uncomplicated otitis externa. The use of systemic antimicrobials to treat AOE has not been found to be beneficial and is associated with adverse side effects, and development of resistance. AOE can be complicated by spread to the pinna or present in an immunocompromised patient. The evidence for topical drops alone is advised for uncomplicated AOE in otherwise healthy patients whilst oral antibiotics may be required if it is not a straightforward case of AOE. Once the patient has been referred then;

1. Meticulous and, if needed, repeated aural toilet, paying particular attention to the antero-inferior meatal recess.

2. Splinting open the meatus. The two recommended choices are 12 millimetre ribbon gauze, impregnated with an anti-bacterial/fungal and steroid cream of choice eg. Trimovate, or a Pope's

sponge otowick onto which eardrops containing an antibiotic and steroid mixture are applied. Splinting will be necessary when there is EAM oedema preventing an adequate view of the tympanic membrane on otoscopy implying that ear drops will not reach the deeper recesses of the ear canal. The dressing should be changed at least every 48 hours until the canal swelling has settled sufficiently to allow any applied drops to reach the whole of the EAC, including the antero-inferior recess, directly

3. Analgesia is also an important part of the management of AOE as it can be particularly painful.

4. Patients should be taught how to correctly administer their topical drops. The patient should lie on their side with the affected ear facing up and administer drops until the ear canal is full. The patient should remain on their side for 3-5 minutes. Gentle movement of the pinna helps the drops move to the affected area and can remove air pockets

3. The ears should be kept scrupulously dry until resolution. Swimming is inadvisable and precautions should be taken when bathing to prevent water entering the ear canal.

It takes three months after resolution of the infection has been achieved for new skin to migrate to replace all the skin of the ear canal. The ear must be kept dry during this time to prevent recurrence.

Follow-up and aftercare

Active treatment should continue for at least one week after resolution because of the tendency to recurrence particularly in fungal infection. Itchy reactive conditions may benefit from a course of

Beclomethasone eardrops. Solution of Aluminium Acetate or Acetic Acid ear spray is recommended in patients with chronic otitis externa after the acute infection has been eradicated.

The most important advice is to keep the ear dry and not to scratch it.

NICE

National Institute for Health and Care Excellence (NICE) has produced clinical knowledge summaries on otitis externa which has recommended topical treatment as a first line since 2010. They recommend topical acetic acid 2% as a first line for mild acute otitis externa and topical antibiotics, with or without a corticosteroid, as a first line in more severe cases. NICE also recommend dry swabbing or microsuction to aid clearing of the external ear canal and advising patients to keep the ear dry and avoid inserting cotton buds into the ear canal.

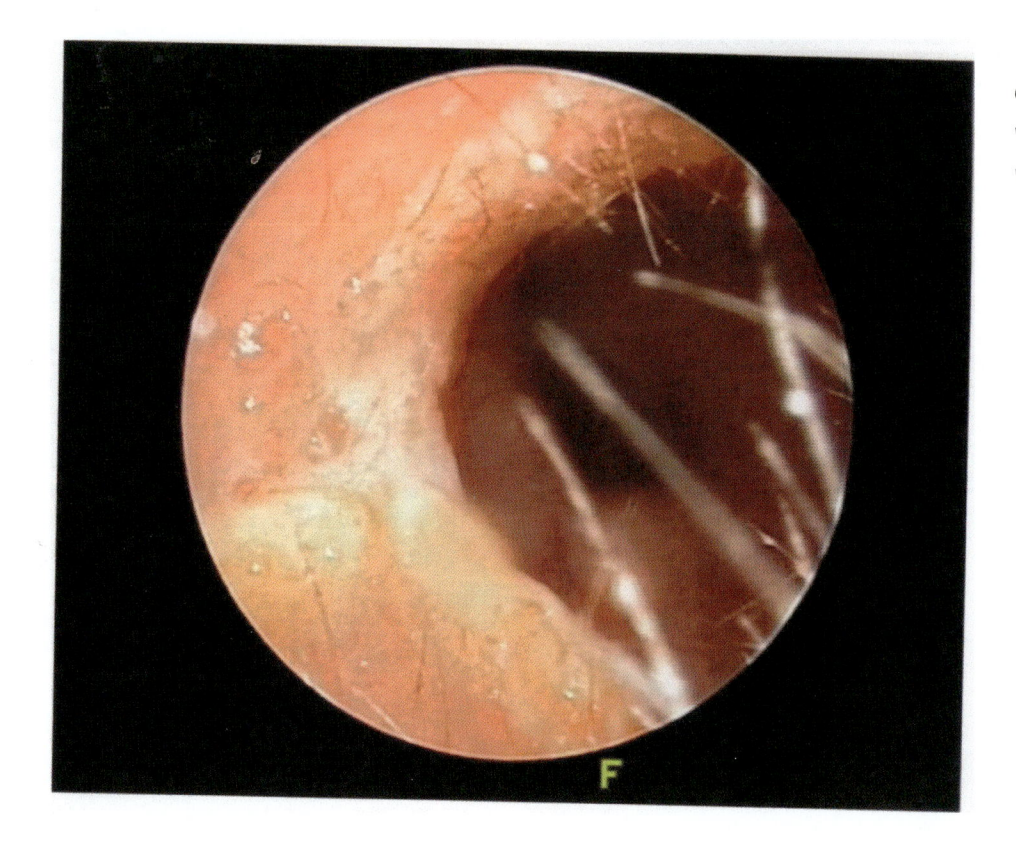

Otitis externa and a very itchy ear with a watery discharge

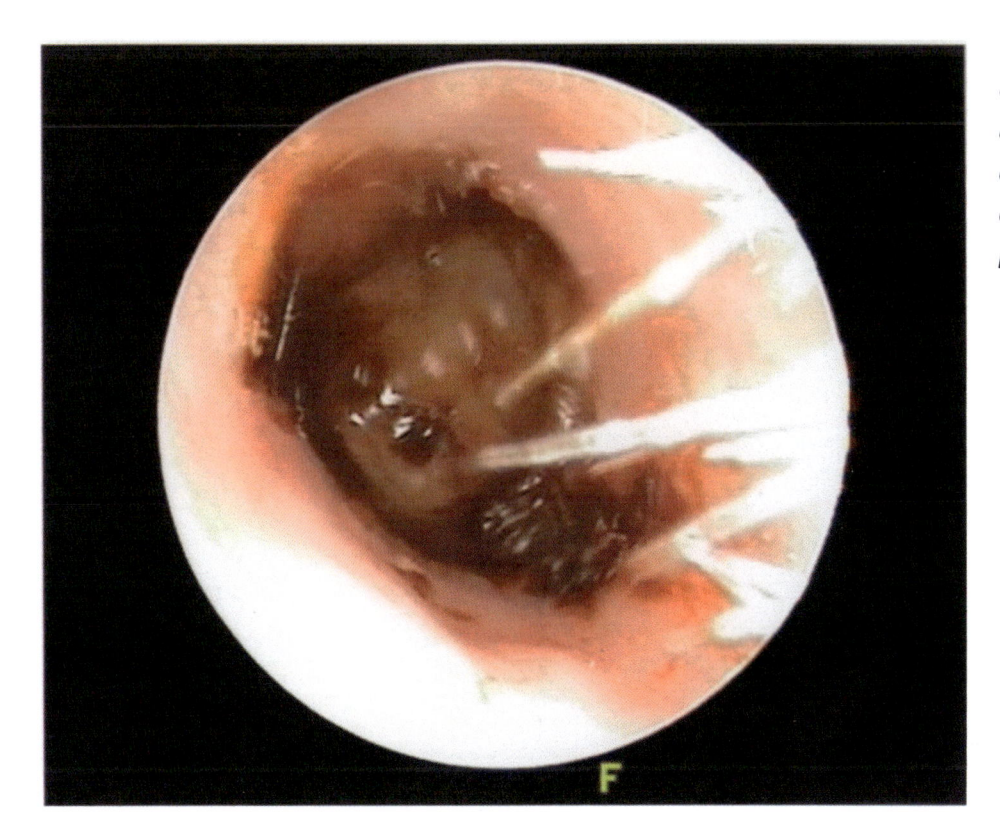

Chronic otitis externa with debris pushed down by the patient cleaning

NECROTISING OTITIS EXTERNA

This is an otitis externa that progresses to an osteomyelitis. Initially it involves the tympanic plate, which is across the floor of the bony ear canal, but may spread to involve the skull base. It is most common after middle age and in diabetics and is usually caused by P. aeruginosa. The overwhelming symptom is a constant deep otalgia and it may cause 7-12th cranial nerve palsies, meningitis, sigmoid sinus thrombosis, brain abscess and death.

The condition should be suspected in a patient with granulation tissue deep in the external meatus that does not settle with the usual treatment. The diagnosis is often not considered until cranial nerve palsy has developed. When such a patient develops facial nerve palsy the differential diagnosis is between Acute Suppurative Otitis Media (where the palsy is almost always secondary to a dehiscent horizontal portion of the facial nerve), Chronic Suppurative Otitis Media, Necrotising Otitis Externa and Carcinoma.

Histological and microbiological examination of the granulation tissue and a high definition CT scan of the temporal bone are required to make the diagnosis.

Treatment

Intravenous antibiotics as determined by the culture and sensitivity results are used. The dose and duration of treatment is decided by monitoring clinical response but often therapy has to be continued for months. Even with aggressive treatment there is still a significant mortality risk.

3 MIDDLE EAR CONDITIONS

Ear Drum and Middle Ear

The eardrum is a circle of thin skin about 8-9mm (one third of an inch) in diameter. Despite its name it is not flat like the skin of a drum but is slightly conical with the curved sides sloping inwards. The eardrum has three layers. The outer layer, in contact with the deep ear canal, is covered with a thin layer of skin. The inner layer, which is in continuity with the lining of the middle ear, consists of rather flat cells that have the ability to transform into the type of cells that line the nose and sinuses and produce mucus. The middle layer of the eardrum is very important and consists of elastic fibres arranged both like the spokes of a wheel [radial fibres] and in circles [circumferential fibres] so that this layer is like a sprung trampoline net. The major portion of the eardrum is tense and absorbs sound [Pars tensa]. The small upper portion of the membrane is more floppy because the fibres of the middle layer are not organized in regular patterns and this region is called the Pars flaccida. The middle ear itself [mesotympanum] lies deep to the eardrum and is an air-filled space that holds three small bones [ossicles] that connect the eardrum to the inner ear. The aditus (opening) is the junction between the upper part of the middle ear (attic or epitympanum) and the air cells of the mastoid.

Middle ear conditions and operations

Cholesteatoma

Cholesteatoma is a collection of "bad skin" (migrating keratinising squamous epithelium) trapped within the middle ear or mastoid. It is a common and potentially dangerous condition. The single most important fact about the skin of the eardrum is that in health it migrates from the centre of the drum outwards along the external ear canal, carrying keratin and wax debris with it. Therefore this skin is self-cleaning .The skin of the eardrum can fairly easily get misplaced and find itself in the middle ear. This can arise from problems in childhood when the Eustachian tube fails to function normally and results in reduced pressures in the middle ear and mastoid. The normal air-pressure in the ear canal then pushes the eardrum skin to retract into the middle ear as a "retraction pocket". This is made easier if middle ear infections have damaged and thinned the membrane so that it loses its resilience. At first the eardrum skin is able to migrate out of the shallow pocket, but if the pocket becomes too deep then the skin is unable to grow around the edge of the pocket and the surface layers of dead skin begin to accumulate. This accumulation of dead skin forces the underlying live skin cells to expand so that layer upon layer of dead cells accumulate and are surrounded by a very thin layer of still living and actively growing eardrum skin. The epithelium eventually loses its capacity to migrate out of the pocket and is trapped. The pocket fills with epithelial debris, which in turn becomes infected and further expands under tension. As it expands the isthmus tends to narrow, compounding the problem and continuing the cycle. As it enlarges the cholesteatoma erodes the structures it encounters, especially bone. This damages the ossicles as well as exposing the inner ear, the facial nerve and the meninges of the brain.

The contents of the cholesteatoma have no blood supply and become easily infected by any bacteria that happen to be around. Skin can also be implanted or migrate around the rim of a Pars tensa pocket or perforation and thus cause a cholesteatoma.

Infection spreads to the various exposed structures. When the cholesteatoma becomes infected foul-smelling pus will be discharged.

The patient complains of deafness and/or foul-smelling discharge. There may be earache. On examination the principal signs are an attic crust, a marginal perforation or a pocket of invading keratin debris. The retraction pocket has become filled with keratin which has turned brown. This resembles wax, but is not. In the three previous images the eardrum, the Pars tensa, is normal. The erosion of bone can lead to reactive polyp formation as the bare bone tries to heal. The polyp is moist and this, in turn, can irritate the deep canal skin with subsequent infection and discharge. Marginal granulations and polyps protruding from the middle ear cleft indicate osteitis and mucosal hyperplasia, respectively. Behind these may lie a cholesteatoma so that micro-suction removal of an attic crust or aural polypectomy may allow the diagnosis to be made

CT scanning of the temporal bone shows a cavity where the affected mastoid bone has been eroded, usually a sclerotic (small mastoid air cells) mastoid is found.

Treatment is usually surgical and aims to make the ear safe. Conservative treatment such as repeated micro-suction can be used in the elderly and infirm or as a temporising means prior to surgery. The incidence is approximately 10 cases per 100 000 population per annum.

The middle ear is surrounded by important structures and the following problems can and do arise:

- Deafness can be due to damage in the bones in the middle ear but can also be due to erosion of the inner ear (labyrinth) which is usually associated with dizziness because of damage to the balance portions of the inner ear.
- The facial nerve which supplies the muscles of facial expression runs through the middle ear and invasion of this by cholesteatoma can cause a facial palsy. Above the middle ear is the brain and invasion of this by the cholesteatoma can cause major neurological conditions including epilepsy and even death. However, the usual way in which cholesteatoma makes its presence known is with a foul smelling discharge secondary to infection of the masses of dead skin.

AURAL CARE

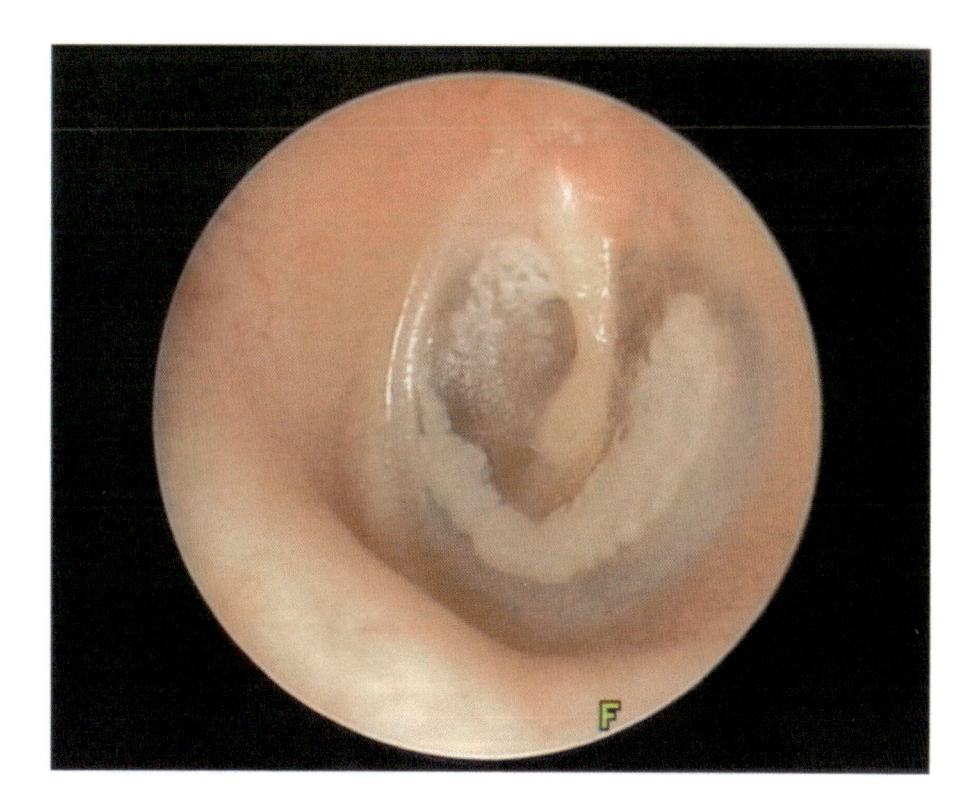

*Horseshoe shaped tympanosclerosis in left ear from childhood grommet. This is **not** cholesteatoma*

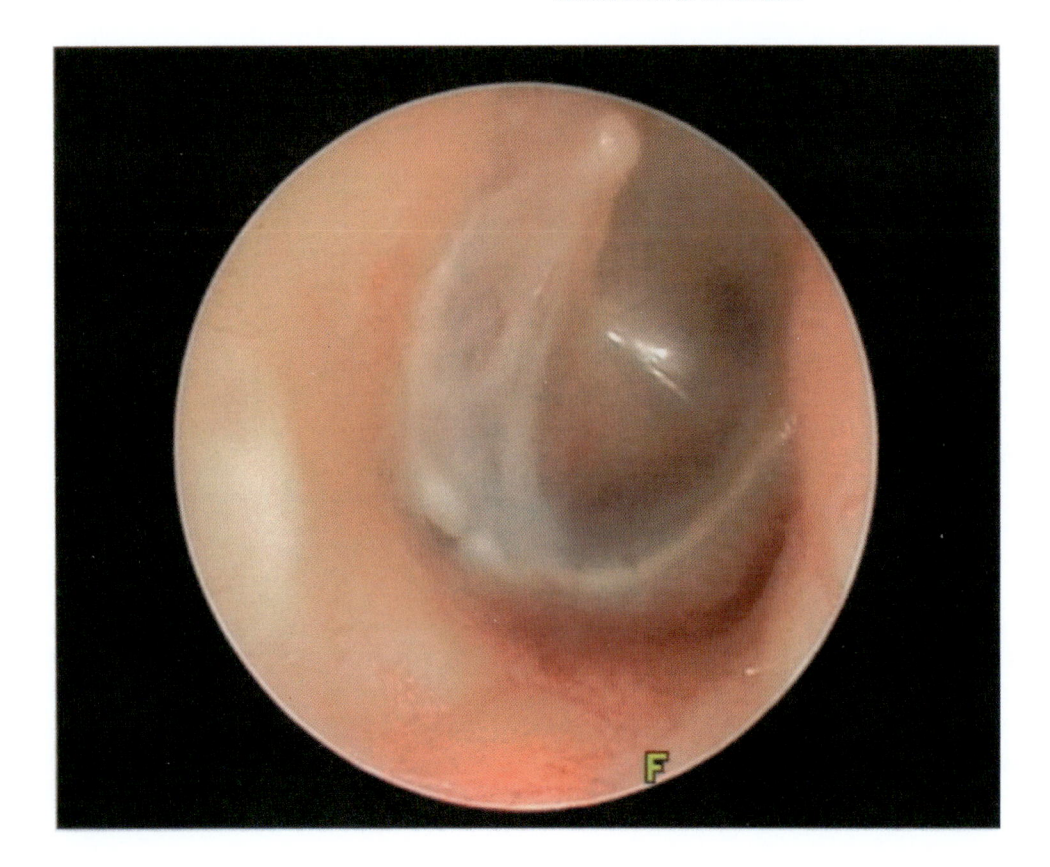

Right ear drum with the annular ligament disrupted 20 years after stapes surgery

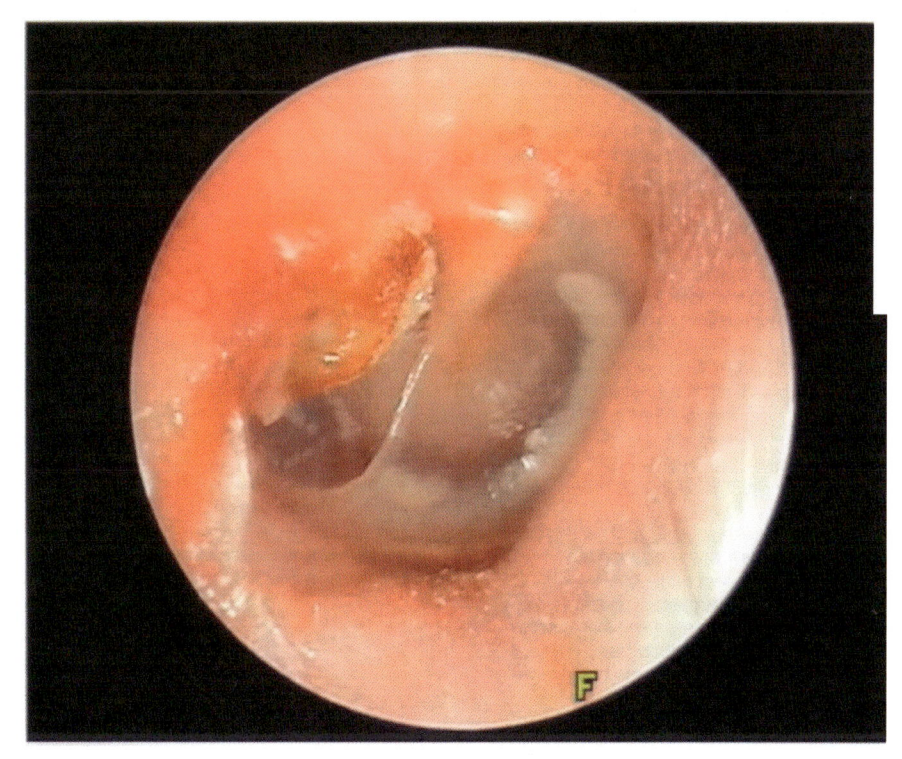

Right ear with pars tensa retraction pocket and cholesteatoma deep to this.

Retraction Pocket

A retraction pocket arises when the middle ear pressure is negative compared to the surrounding air. In an otherwise normal tympanic membrane it is the Pars flaccida that retracts because of its greater flexibility secondary to the structure of its middle layer.

If the Pars tensa has been previously perforated and healed then the middle layer is generally absent, so this will retract if there is pressure imbalance (or indeed balloon outwards if there is a positive middle ear pressure).

The use of the word *pocket* implies some depth to the structure rather than a slight retraction. If the migratory skin of the pocket, flaccida or tensa, can still migrate outwards then the pocket is termed "self - cleaning". If not then then dead skin (keratin) will accumulate and a cholesteatoma may form. Published evidence suggests that perhaps 16% of retraction pockets develop into a cholesteatoma. When a retraction pocket is found on examination, the full extent of the retraction pocket should be ascertained to assess the presence and extent of any disease such as cholesteatoma.

Eustachian tube dysfunction

To enable effective hearing, air is needed either side of the tympanic membrane in order to facilitate sound collection and its transference onwards to the inner ear.

The middle ear is lined with tissue containing mucus-producing glands and a surface covered with flexible cilia (hairs) again not dissimilar to those in the nose. As such the middle ear is an air filled space with tissue capable of producing debris from the dead surface cells and mucus from the glands.

This leads to two problems. First is clearing the debris and mucus. The second is a more subtle but very important problem. Oxygen is absorbed from the air in the middle ear into the blood vessels running through its lining in much the same way that oxygen is absorbed in the lungs. Some carbon dioxide is given off into the air in the middle ear, but with a dysfunctional Eustachian tube, over the passage of time, the effect is a drop in middle ear pressure as the oxygen is removed. With atmospheric pressure outside the eardrum, something has to give and the only thing that can move is the eardrum. This would be pushed inwards by the external pressure and would stop normal function. Eventually the whole middle ear would collapse and a significant hearing loss would develop.

When working properly, the Eustachian tube prevents both these problems. This tube runs forwards and inwards from the front wall of the middle ear to open into the back of the nasal cavity above the soft palate (the nasopharynx). The end nearer the nose is soft and flexible and opens on swallowing or yawning. Although the precise mechanism is unclear, this tubal opening allows enough air up into the middle ear to replenish it and keep the middle ear pressures close to atmospheric. It has been calculated that only one or two mls. of air per ear per day – that is less than half a teaspoon of air - are necessary to maintain proper ventilation of the middle ear, but without this the middle ear fails.

The Eustachian tube is also the conduit along which the cilia move the normal mucus produced in the middle ear to the back of the nose where in turn it is swallowed. This thin film of mucus, carrying the debris produced in the middle ear, is moved along the floor of the Eustachian tube with air passing above it to reach the middle ear from the nose. Thus, the two functions of ventilation and self-cleansing are achieved when the system is working properly. Unfortunately, in man the mechanism is rather fragile and often fails to function adequately, possibly because of the shape and elongation of the skull base needed to accommodate the large brain,

There is also an extension of the air filled spaces of the middle ear backwards into the mastoid bone, which if you put your hand to the back of the ear can be felt as a rounded bump. This should be hollow with the air filled spaces broken up by small and incomplete bony partitions. The average mastoid has an air volume of about 15-20 mls and this helps buffer pressure changes in the middle ear and reduce adverse effects on the tympanic membrane. Individuals with small mastoid air spaces seem to be at a much greater risk of developing middle ear and mastoid disease. Whether it is the middle ear and mastoid disease that causes the failure of the mastoid to develop or whether the small size reduces the buffering power and therefore causes the development of disease is yet to be fully answered. The likely answer, though, is that it will be a bit of both.

OPERATIONS

Mastoidectomy

In this operation the diseased and infected tissues are removed leaving a cavity. In a modified radical mastoidectomy there is preservation of as much of the non-diseased middle ear contents as is possible. The cavity may be repaired or obliterated and the ossicles replaced either at the time of the mastoidectomy or at a second sitting. There may be a cavity that needs cleaning for the rest of the patient's life. Although the mastoidectomy will usually give the patient a safe ear, this may be at the price of a hearing loss.

Tympanoplasty

The operation of tympanoplasty is designed to reconstruct the middle ear and close a hole in the ear drum to allow swimming or to improve hearing. It must be carried out on a safe ear, preferably a dry one. It involves the repair to the drum perforation and the reconstruction of the defects in the ossicular chain. Fascia, for instance, from the temporalis muscle, which is readily accessible above the pinna, is used for the graft to repair the drum. A bed is first prepared for the fascia by de-epithelialisation of the perforation's edges, so ensuring that skin cannot grow into the middle ear. Some types of tympanoplasty will include ossicular reconstruction as well as drum repair.

Tympanoplasty is described as either central or marginal. Central Perforation need not be in the centre of the tympanic membrane. It is a perforation that has a rim (however narrow) of normal drum between the edge of the perforation and the bony annulus. In Marginal Tympanoplasty there is no drum between it and bony annulus, and it extends to the bony margin. The distinction between the two types of perforation is important because marginal perforations are more likely to produce choleastomas especially posterior marginal perforations.

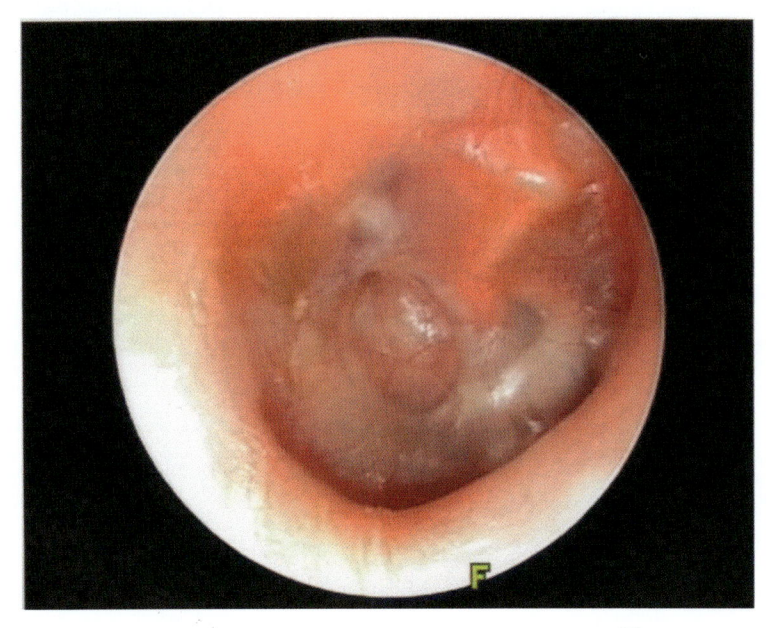

Previous tympanoplasty for cholesteatoma with no signs of recurrence

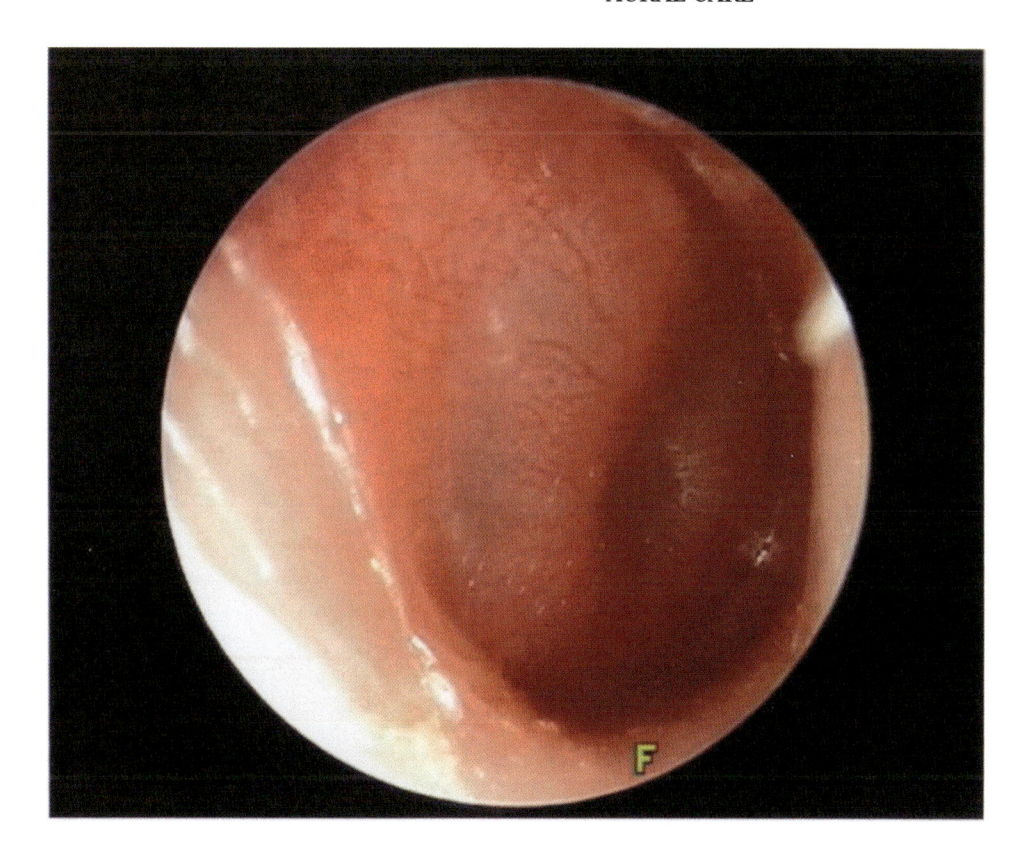

Bulging right ear with glue ear. Note the "sea shore" effect on the posterior part of the ear canal

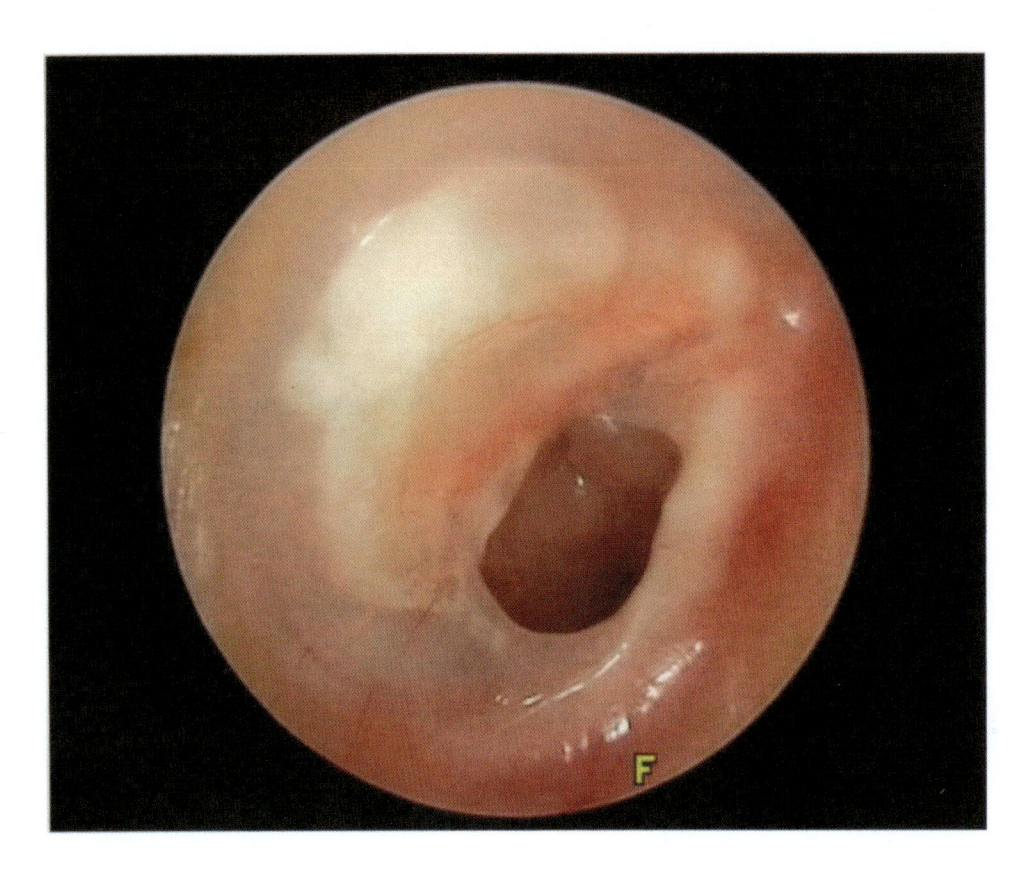

Anterior perforation in right ear with posterior tympanosclerotic plaque

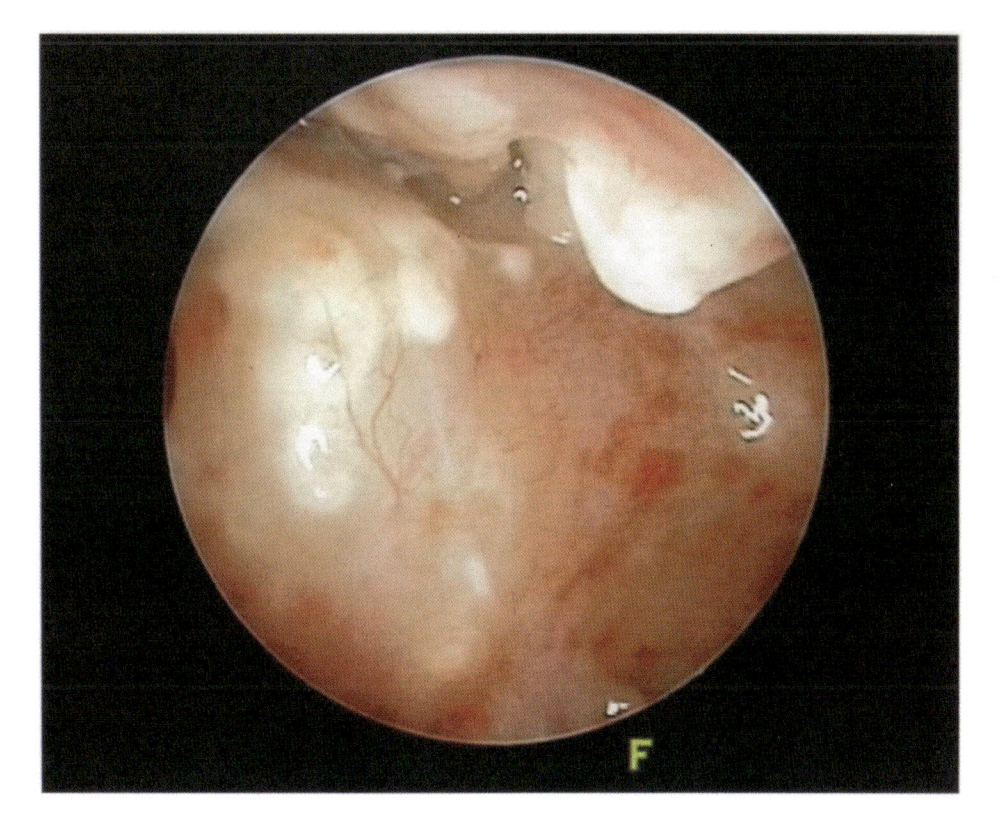

View through a perforation showing tympanosclerosis of the middle ear fixing of the ossicles

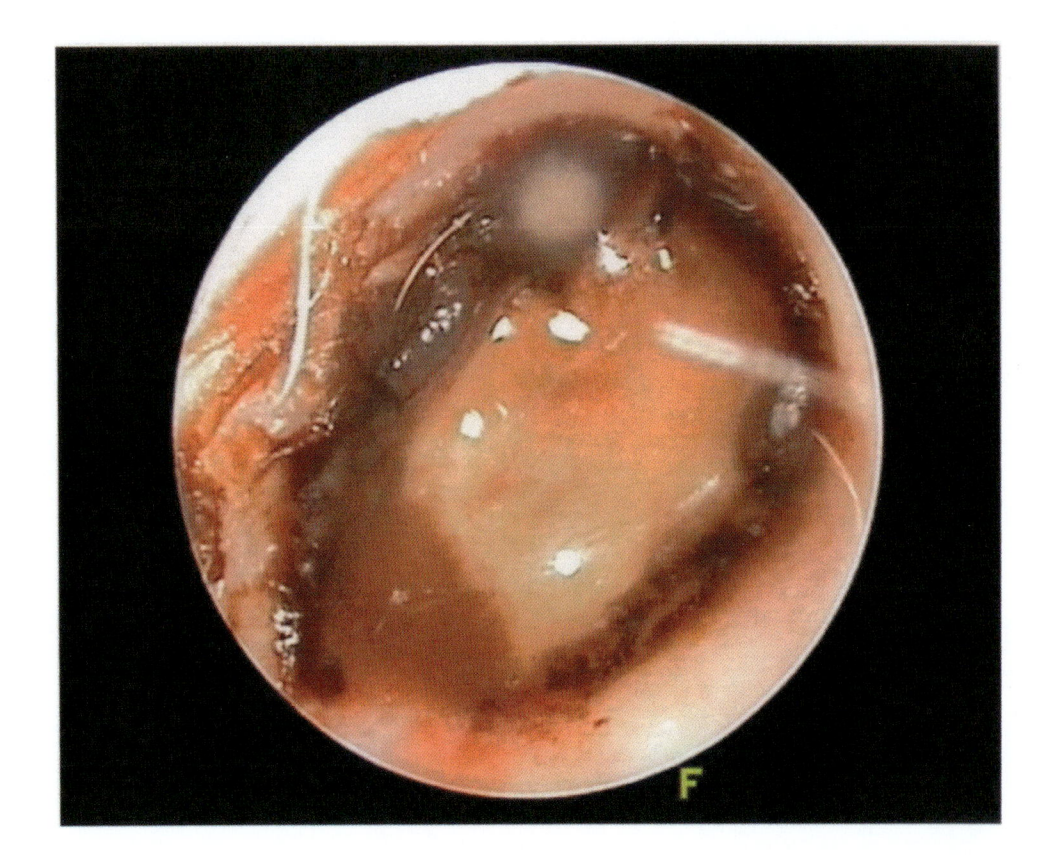

Wax and debris in chronically discharging ear with previous mastoid surgery

AURAL CARE

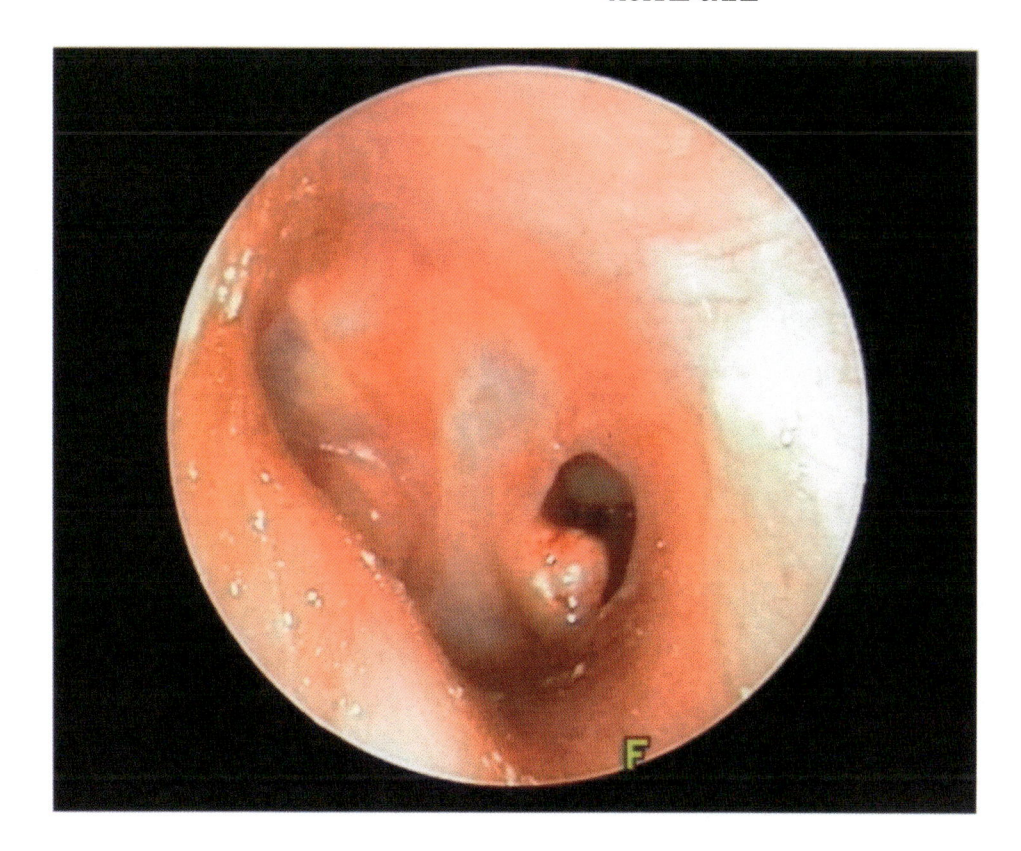

Failed tympanoplasty The displaced graft can be seen through the residual perforation

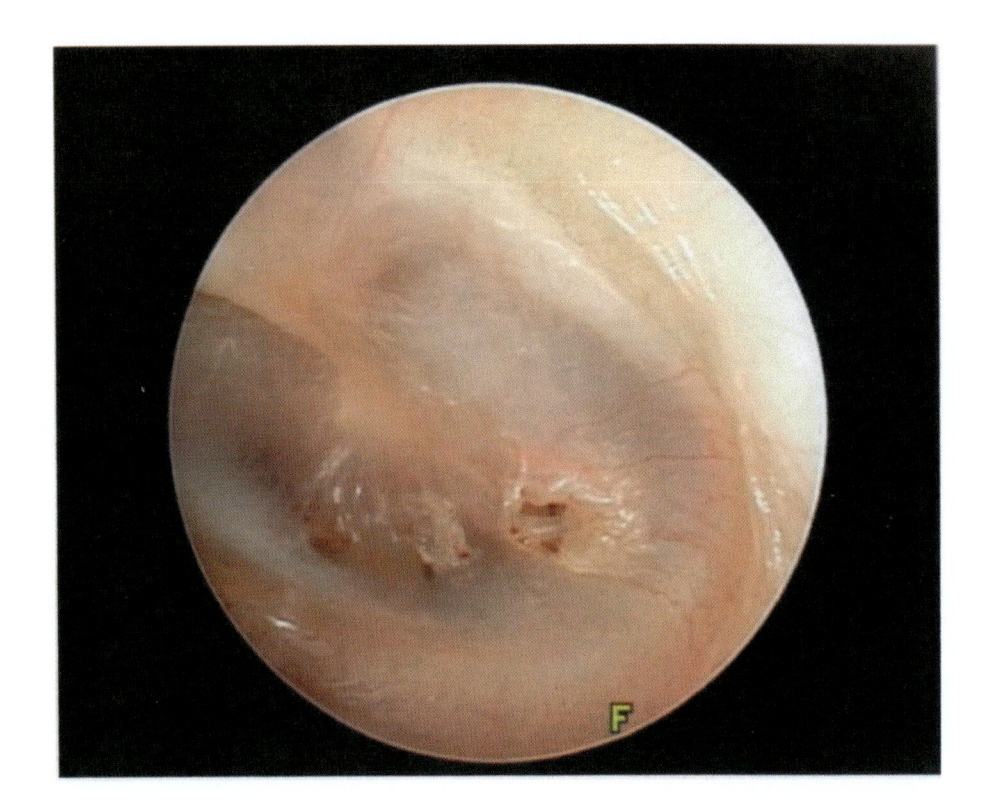

Traumatic Perforation two weeks after being hit on ear

4 INNER EAR CONDITIONS

INNER EAR

The inner ear has the three symptoms of sensory neural deafness, vertigo and tinnitus which are to some extent beyond the scope of this text. There is one otological emergency, however, Idiopathic Sudden Sensory Neural Hearing Loss (SSNHL) that may come to the aural care nurse and should be recognised.

Idiopathic Sudden Sensory Neural Hearing Loss

This occurs in 1 in 5,000 of the population every year. It is commonly misdiagnosed as wax or glue ear in General Practice. A careful history and examination including using tuning forks will make the diagnosis. The treatment is steroids. SSNHL can be defined as a sensorineural hearing loss of 30 dB or more in at least three contiguous frequencies, developing within a three-day period *(Remember "30-3-3")*. The peak age is in the 50-59 year group with a range of 10-79 and an equal sex distribution. It is a condition of unknown cause with a number of postulated theories as to its cause including vascular, viral and cochlear membrane breaks. A percentage of cases of sudden hearing loss are caused by acoustic neuroma and more rarely lyme disease or syphilis.

There is a high spontaneous resolution rate in sudden sensorineural hearing loss with up to 65% of patients having a recovery to functional hearing without medical treatment. The presence of vertigo may be a poor prognostic sign. It is common practice in the UK to prescribe a short course of oral steroids (eg prednisolone 60mg daily, reducing over ten days) for SSNHL.

Management in the first instance is aimed at investigating identifiable causes for SSNHL and treating them as appropriate. Therapies in SSNHL are aimed at improving cochlear microcirculation and thus oxygenation and steroids improve the cochlear blood flow as well as their many other effects.

It is also useful to remember that unilateral or asymmetric inner ear symptoms should be scanned using an MRI scanner to exclude an Acoustic Neuroma.

The diagnosis and management of Acoustic Neuroma, or as it should really be called Vestibular Schwannoma (it grows from the vestibular nerve sheath rather than the acoustic nerve),are beyond the scope this text.

5 OTORRHOEA

Otorrhoea is the discharge of material from the ear. It is both a symptom and a sign but it is not a diagnosis.

Otitis externa and suppurative otitis media are the commonest diseases causing this problem. Other causes include: wax, debris, blood (acute otitis media, trauma, neoplasm), and CSF (usually following a fracture). In some forms of otitis externa the "modified sweat glands that produce wax" have changed to produce a discharge that is like sweat. It may be profuse and cause the patients to complain and clean their ears. It may even stain the cotton bud used pink.

Clinical features

The character of the discharge depends on (and therefore gives clues to) its source.

1. External ear

    There are no mucinous glands in the external canal. Acute inflammatory conditions of the external canal therefore tend to produce a watery, serous exudate or transudate. In addition, they tend to provoke a hyperkeratosis, more skin formation. This combination generally leads to soggy white debris collecting in the canal and a thin white watery discharge from the ear. The cardinal symptom of otitis externa is itchiness in addition to the discharge, pain and tenderness. The external canal may also be the subject of trauma, which may lead to bleeding from the ear.

2. Middle ear

The middle ear cleft is well endowed with mucous glands. Thus, if there is a mucoid component to the discharge it usually arises from the middle ear via a perforation of the tympanic membrane. Trapped keratin is offensive; if a cholesteatoma becomes infected the discharge tends to be particularly unpleasant and once smelt is never forgotten. A serosanguinous discharge is common with chronic otitis media when the middle ear mucosa has become granular and polypoid. There is glandular hyperplasia and there may be blood as the mucosa bleeds easily. Blood stained discharge is also a feature of carcinoma of the middle ear. Chronic otitis media is not typically characterized by pain, so in patients where chronic otorrhoea becomes painful and fails to respond to the usual conservative measures, it is wise to consider a carcinoma.

3. Cerebrospinal fluid

CSF rarely discharges from the ears spontaneously but may do so following skull base surgery or more commonly trauma, when it will develop in about 5 % of cases. In both cases the fluid may initially be mixed with blood and may be recognized by the halo sign in which there is a clear ring of moisture surrounding the blood after absorption on to blotting paper or the patient's pillow. This is due to the faster diffusion of the less viscous CSF. Differentiation of CSF from thin serous discharge from a middle ear cavity may be more difficult but can be done by confirming the presence of B2-transferrin in CSF. If the tympanic membrane is intact CSF may still leak from the ear should there be a fracture in the roof of the ear canal. Otherwise it will pass down the Eustachian tube and become evident as rhinorrhoea or post- nasal drip.

Management

Optimum management depends on making an accurate diagnosis. Although the history will give many clues, the diagnosis is usually not made until the tympanic membrane has been visualized. This may not be possible at the initial consultation owing to swelling and debris in the external auditory meatus. A swab should be taken for culture and sensitivity (bacteria/fungi). This is especially important in patients who have already been on treatments that have not worked. Any granulation type tissue removed should be sent for histology. The mainstay of therapy is aural toilet, ideally by micro-suction clearance. This enables a thorough assessment, diagnosis of cause, and allows better penetration of any topical treatments.**Treatment**

Treatment will often start on the basis of a best guess diagnosis. This will invariably require attention to the primary or secondary otitis externa by thorough aural toilet and possibly the insertion of a wick. At the time of definitive diagnosis more appropriate treatment can be continued. Treatment of the otitis externa will be sufficient if this is the diagnosis. Middle ear disease will demand treatment on its own merits.

Patients with CSF otorrhoea are at risk of meningitis. Posttraumatic leaks usually resolve spontaneously within a short period but surgical repair will be required if they continue.

6 BEFORE STARTING MICRO-SUCTION

Before starting micro-suction:

- Introduce yourself;

- Position the patient;

- Start with the better ear;

- Inspect the pinna, mastoid and external auditory meatus. Examine the pinna in front and behind for scars, redness, swelling and skin lesions. The mastoid area should be carefully examined for scars, swelling, redness or tenderness. Look for discharge from the external auditory meatus as well as any changes of the skin.

- Methodically examine the tympanic membrane. Insert a suitably sized speculum for insertion into the external canal. To examine the external auditory canal, pull the pinna upwards, outwards and backwards. In young children pull downwards and backwards. Introduce the speculum just past the hairs of the outer canal, but avoid contact with the sensitive bony part of the canal. A good view of the tympanic membrane should then be possible as well as the malleus and the handle of the malleus. Examine all quadrants of the membrane. Look for the light reflex (this is antero-inferior) and is the only part of the ear drum that is perpendicular to the light going in and therefore reflects like a mirror. The ear drum is cone shaped and at an angle of 137 degrees to the ear canal such that the posterior part is much closer to the outside than the anterior part. The long process of the incus is sometimes observed behind and parallel to the handle of the malleus and it is sometimes possible to see it articulate with the head of the stapes.

  Look for a perforation and note its position, size and whether it is central or marginal. Look through any perforation that you may see for the promontory, round window, incudostapedial joint, or some cholesteatoma. If the patient has had mastoid surgery assess access (meatoplasty size and height of the facial ridge) and decide if the cavity is healthy or not.

- You may also need to check the Facial nerve, do tuning fork tests and consider a Fistula test and, if audiology is not available, do free-field voice tests.

  The Rinne test compares the loudness of the tuning fork by air conduction or bone conduction (on the mastoid process). The normal response is to hear the sound as louder with air conduction and is referred to as a Rinne positive. A positive response will also occur with a sensorineural hearing loss. A negative response (Rinne negative) will occur if there is a conductive loss of greater than 20 dB or if there is a severe sensorineural hearing loss. The former is referred to as a true-negative Rinne and the latter as a false negative as the bone conduction is really being heard in the opposite ear through bone conduction. The opposite ear has to be masked with noise to see if it is a false negative.

You can perform a fistula test by applying tragal pressure and looking for movement of the eyes away from that side.

Free-field speech tests are done by asking the patient to repeat double figure numbers or bi-syllabic words spoken with a whispered voice, conversation voice and, if needs be, shouted voice at 60 cm from the ear. The non-test ear is masked by pressing the tragus backwards and rotating it with the index finger. The patient sits side-on so that lip reading is not possible.

7 WAX

This chapter is an example of evidence-based practice from discussions of this problem. It also demonstrates to aural care nurses, especially advanced nurse practitioners, how they can formulate their evidence-based practice.

Categories of Evidence

1. Evidence from meta-analysis of randomised controlled trials or from at least one randomised controlled trial;
2. Evidence from at least one controlled study without randomisation or at least one other type of quasi- experimental study;
3. Evidence from non-experimental descriptive studies, such as comparative studies, correlation studies and case control studies;
4. Evidence from expert committee reports or opinions and/or clinical experience of respected authorities.

Strength of Recommendations

A. Directly based on category 1 evidence;

B. Directly based on category 2 evidence or extrapolated recommendation from category 1 evidence;
C. Directly based on category 3 evidence or extrapolated recommendation from category 1 or 2 evidence;
D. Directly based on category 4 evidence or extrapolated recommendation from category 1, 2 or 3 evidence.

WAX REMOVAL - IS IT NECESSARY?

Wax is a normal physiological substance and should only be removed if it is causing the patient symptoms (Level A recommendation) or if it prevents inspection of the tympanic membrane (Level D recommendation)

Rationale

Wax removal has been shown to improve hearing in those patients with impacted wax. Memel et al (2002) demonstrated a mean improvement in hearing of 6.9 decibels after wax removal. A postal survey by Sharp et al (1990) concluded that removal of wax improved patients' hearing by a mean of 5.45 decibels. Both studies indicate a clinically significant improvement in hearing as a result of wax removal. Patients seek wax removal for a range of symptoms including hearing problems, blocked ears, noises in the ears, itchy ears, dizziness and ear pain (Sharp et al 1990; Browning 2001; Memel et al 2002). These symptoms are not easy to quantify and objectively assess.

One randomised controlled trial (Memel et al 2002) looked at patients' subjective benefits from wax removal. Patients' subjective reports of their change in symptoms included:

1) Difficulty hearing on the phone: 75% experienced improvement.
2) Pain: 70% experienced improvement.
3) Blocked ears: 62 % experienced improvement.
4) Difficulty hearing one-to-one: 61 % experienced improvement.
5) Difficulty hearing in a group: 55% experienced improvement.
6) Noises: 49% experienced improvement.
7) Dizziness: 48% experienced improvement.
8) Itchy ears: 39% experienced improvement.

Objective measurements are based on a category 1 evidence paper and a postal survey; these two papers provided consistent evidence that wax removal improved hearing. Subjective reports as to improvement in hearing and blocked ears correlated well with objective measurement

WAX SOFTNERS - WHICH CERUMINOLYTIC?

A ceruminolytic should be advised if the wax is hard and impacted. Sodium bicarbonate is the ceruminolytic of choice in the acute phase, the optimum time for use being 5 days. Olive oil is the lubricant of choice for chronic problems (Level D recommendation).

Rationale

The literature search revealed no objective, unbiased, randomised controlled trials as to the best wax softener. Browning (2001) details this lack of evidence: use of a wax softener versus no treatment reduced the risk of impaction if it was used for five days. A ceruminolytic should soften, loosen, liquefy and disintegrate wax. The survey conducted by Sharp (1990) indicated that the most commonly advised ceruminolytic was olive oil.

Hawke (2002) provided in-vitro evidence that the use of sodium bicarbonate and water are better than oil. He found that the chemical composition of wax responded better to aqueous solutions such as water and sodium bicarbonate as they provided better breakdown of the wax. Oil based solutions only lubricated the wax. In-vitro studies proved that olive oil appeared to be totally ineffective in dispersing earwax: water was more effective. Eeekhof et al (2001) in a prospective randomised trial concluded that water, used for 15 minutes prior to syringing in patients with persistent wax, worked well in daily practice with real patients.

Of the proprietary brands, Sharp et al (1990) found that Cerumol was the drug of choice given by doctors. However a large multi-centre trial found Exterol to be significantly more effective than Cerumol (Fahmy 1982). Studies have revealed sodium bicarbonate to be more effective than oil, if instilled correctly. The BNF states that both preparations are equally safe and inexpensive.

The joint Formulary Committee feels proprietary brands are less suitable for prescribing and should not be the first drug of choice (BNF 2002), as they may cause irritation and inflammation to the external ear canal.

There was no level 1 evidence that wax softeners work better than a placebo. Nevertheless the consensus is that they do.

ASSESSMENT OF SUITABILITY FOR EAR SYRINGING

A full otological history and examination should be undertaken prior to syringing the ear.

Check for contraindications to minimise complications.

- Patient history as to previous and current ear problems and conditions - read patient notes and ask patient
- End-aural and post auricular examination for signs of an incision, which would indicate previous surgery; skin problems indicating otitis externa, severe pain on manipulation of pinna
- Otoscopy to assess wax and any stenosis of the ear canal, or mucopurulent discharge in ear canal, which usually signifies middle ear disease
- Document the findings in a structured format
- If in doubt about suitability ***DO NOT SYRINGE*** (Level D recommendation).

Rationale

It has been acknowledged in the literature that complications do arise from ear syringing (Sharp et al 1990; Price 1997; Blake et al 1998; Grossan 1996). However, the incidence is unknown.

Evidence found due to litigation claims points to the need for accurate otological assessment. Practitioners should know the contra-indications to ear syringing in order to decrease complications. Blake et al (1998) when dealing with litigation claims during the period 1992-1993 reported that, out of 47 accepted ear syringing claims, 17 ears were syringed with the patients having a clear otological history, while the others had persistent otitis externa. It was concluded in general that the practice documentation was inadequate and often markedly different from the claimants' versions.

This was confirmed by Price (1997), who says that the main cause for complications that the Medical Defence Union found were failure to take a full history or examine the ear, so the contraindications to syringing were not found. 69% of practitioners who were involved in litigation were found to have poor record keeping and history taking was not documented . Practice falls short of what is ideal.

Complications found in Sharpe et al's survey (1990) indicated that 38% of the GPs reviewed had encountered complications. The commonest was a failure to remove wax.

The next highest complication was a perforated tympanic membrane. The evidence provided by Price (1997) showed that the most common adverse outcome was a perforated tympanic membrane, which happened in 35% of the claims. Evidence provided in a Level 2 study by Vibeke et al (1995) who performed in-vitro syringing showed the pressure developed in the external auditory meatus was insufficient to rupture a normal tympanic membrane. They concluded that if a perforation arose it was due to the fact that the tympanic membrane was not normal prior to the procedure. Weakening occurs as a consequence of a healed perforation, recurrent infections, otitis media with effusion. Grommets may extrude leaving a thinner tympanic membrane segment. Unhealed perforations are a marked contra-indication to syringing (Blake et al 1998).

Evidence strongly points to the fact that complications are avoided by obtaining a full otological history and examining the ear for prior pathology (Grossan 1998). Collection of data in a structured format will enable consideration of clinical factors that may impact on the need to syringe ears. If the patient gives a poor history and the tympanic membrane cannot be examined due to wax impaction, and if there is no previous documented visual examination of the eardrum available, do not syringe the ear.

Contraindications

- History of perforated ear drum Previous or pending ear surgery
- Previous or current history of ear disease Otitis externa
- Previous injury or a stated aversion to ear syringing
- Only one hearing ear
- Stenosed ear canals, which may be a result of infections or bony exostosis
- Foreign bodies, sharp or hygroscopic in nature
- Known inner ear disturbance causing severe vertigo

SYRINGING - METAL OR ELECTRIC?

There is no evidence that electric is better or worse than the metal syringe. The most important factor when using either metal or electric syringe is that the person using it is trained and experienced to operate it.

Other factors include:
- The syringing equipment is properly maintained
- The syringe is assembled correctly prior to use and the nozzle is firmly attached
- Verbal consent is obtained
- Correct technique is used
- Procedure is stopped if patient experiences any problems
- Check ears after syringing to see if wax is removed, and that no complications have arisen
- Dry any excess water from the ear
- Document the procedure, noting which syringe used, attempts and any adverse problems during procedure
- (Level D recommendation)

Rationale

No evidence was found that the metal is better or worse than the electric ear syringe. The randomised trial (Memel et al 2002) looking at the effectiveness of ear syringing in general practice used both the metal and electric syringe with no detrimental effects noted with either. In 1998 a study by Kent found that nurses were divided in their use of ear syringing equipment: they made their choice on the confidence they had in using the syringe and the results obtained and thus their choice was not based on research. No papers were found relating to metal ear syringe versus electric ear syringe.

Vibeke et al (1995) provided good evidence that normal pressure produced by the metal ear syringe is insufficient to rupture a healthy eardrum. They concluded that they could confirm that ear syringing in general was a safe practice. Blake et al (1998) in their litigation claims found that the evidence indicates that the metal syringe will not perforate a healthy eardrum if used properly.

The main evidence found points to poor maintenance and assembly of equipment prior to syringing. A Medical Devices Agency safety notice (SN 9807) issued in February 1998 in regards to the *Propulse* suggested that the low and top end stops should be checked before every use, as excessive force on the output control can break the end stop and cause damage in the ear. No notices have been declared on the updated model, the *Propulse II*.

A report by Dinsdale (1991) discusses a patient receiving injuries in the external ear canal with a dental tip from an electric syringe. Price (1997) quotes one incidence of negligence due to poor assembly of equipment: "Nozzle of a metal syringe came adrift during ear syringing causing a perforation". The metal syringe must be lubricated properly and nozzle firmly attached prior to each syringing. The *Propulse II* in its manufacturer's guidelines indicates the need to attach a jet tip. It also has available for use a disposable angled jet tip, for one use only, and again care in assembly is required.

Bapat (2001) provides further evidence that complications arise despite no contraindications, but they report a case of a patient suffering audio-vestibular damage due to the nozzle of a syringe being inserted too far down the external auditory canal and traumatising the ossicles and fracturing the stapes bone. Blake et al (1995) support this when discussing the technique of syringing. They stress that the nozzle should not be inserted too deep into the canal and that the pinna should be pulled up and back and the syringe directed along the postero-superior canal wall, so that the syringe is not pointed directly at the tympanic membrane. Such evidence supports the need for thorough training programmes.

The literature suggests that syringing may precipitate an infection, so the ear should be dried after syringing to remove residual water. The equipment should be decontaminated appropriately as per manufacturers 'instructions. Manual ear syringing equipment should not be stored wet. *Propulse* manufacturers' instructions stress that water at the end of the day should be discarded as any left could build up bacteria. including pseudomonas, a common reason for patients requiring treatment for otitis externa. No studies were available, however, to provide evidence as to the incidence of this. Whilst there is no evidence that wax syringing in an otherwise normal ear causes deafness there are occasional circumstantial case reports of this. It is therefore prudent to warn the patient that unforeseen problems can occur with any procedure and that these could include deafness, dizziness, tinnitus, perforation and infection but that these are very rare.

Summary

Wax should be removed if this is causing the patient symptoms. These symptoms may include difficulty hearing, pain blocked ears, noises, dizziness and itchy ears. Wax softeners can be used for a period of five days, Sodium bicarbonate being the ceruminolytic of choice in the acute phase and olive oil being the lubricant of choice for chronic problems, or if any otitis externa has occurred .

When assessing the suitability for ear syringing and being aware of the contra-indications, ear syringing can be done either with the electric or hand syringe and excess water should be dried away. Documentation is mandatory.

Manual removal is appropriate for patients with contra-indications to syringing. There is no evidence to demonstrate that this is better or worse than syringing in normal patients but in patients with contra-indications to syringing it is the only option available. This is where aural care clinics come in.

8 GUIDELINES

GENERAL GUIDELINES FOR AURAL MICRO-SUCTION

There is little evidence for the treatments once the patient has been sent to the aural care clinic. Here are some examples of protocols that could be used/adapted for your area.

1. **Prior to treatment by a nurse, the nurse must record in the patient's notes:**

   - verbal consent to treatment by the nurse

   - history of past and present ear problems

   - previous and current state of hearing.

   - any relevant past major medical problem (i.e. cardiac, chest, hiatus hernia, arthritis, allergies etc).

   - current medication.

   - any contra-indications to micro-suction: recent vertigo, severe pre-existing pain bleeding, possible/known

- damage to middle ear structures, inability to lie down/lie still recent ear surgery.

2. Examination of the ears

- The nurse introduces him/herself as the person to be giving the treatment

- Patient is asked to lie down on the couch

- Wash hands

- The pinna and surrounding skin are assessed for any swelling, inflammation, tenderness, ulceration, scarring, evidence of previous surgery/treatment

- Document, sign and date findings

- The microscope should be switched on, taking care that the light is not directed at the patient's face

- The speculum with the largest diameter that fits comfortably into the meatus should be used

- Examine the meatus for any narrowing, nodules, redness, dryness, swelling, discharge, cysts, foreign objects, excessive wax.

3. Remember:

- The external ear does not have any mucous glands. Therefore if there is a mucous discharge it must have originated from the middle ear and the patient must have a perforation with underlying middle ear infection or cholesteatoma - **REFER** after cleaning.

- Document, sign and date findings.

- Proceed according to the relevant guidelines, if unsure **REFER** to doctor's clinic.

4. Patient Education

- Inform the patient how to care for ears

- Emphasize importance of and how to keep the ears dry

- Ensure the patient knows how to instil ear drops correctly

- Ensure the patient knows how to obtain further treatment

- Advise against the use of cotton buds

- Advise against non-prescribed 'remedies'

- Discuss effects of lifestyle and stress on aural condition

5. Documentation

Record all

- Observations made

- Treatments given

- Education/information given

- Treatment plan/discharge from clinic/SOS appointment

- Sign, date and time all entries

6. Communication

- Send letter to GP outlining treatment given

- Arrange follow-up appointment

- Explain to patient how to get help in an emergency

- Give written instructions as appropriate.

GUIDELINES FOR THE TREATMENT OF OTITIS EXTERNA OTITIS EXTERNA

Otitis externa is an inflammation of the skin lining the external auditory canal (EAC), sometimes involving the pinna. It can be infective (bacterial, fungal or viral) or reactive (allergy or eczema). It can also occur as an acute episode or be a chronic condition. It is one of the most common ear complaints.

Predisposing factors include:

- Trauma - cotton buds, ear syringing, hearing aids
- Swimming - in susceptible individuals
- Allergy - eczema, dermatitis, dandruff, psoriasis
- Secondary - to middle ear disease

Symptoms

- Itchy, irritation can be unbearable

AURAL CARE

- Discharge
- Deafness - if inflammation has occluded EAC
- Pain - usually only with acute infection
- Narrowed canals - may be tender
- Tender tragus
- Discharge

Remove predisposing factors and treat both infection and any underlying skin disorders.

Initial Consultation

- Examine ear. If able to perform aural suction to remove residual debris, proceed with caution as the ear will be tender and may bleed.
- Take swab for culture and sensitivity

If the meatus is closed due to oedema, a ribbon gauze dressing soaked in a cream antibacterial/fungal/steroid e.g. Trimovate should be inserted to reduce the swelling and relieve inflammation. Change dressing on alternate days until meatus opens, if patient unable to attend or no clinic available a " POPE " wick soaked in Gentisone HC (if patient has no contraindications, see PGD) should be used and the patient advised to apply 3-4 drops 3 times daily directly onto wick for 7 days.

Review Patient 1 week

- Remove the debris and discharge with the suction, look for polyps, crusts and cholesteatoma

- Review swab results

- Local steroid and/or antibiotic drops should be dispensed according to the agreed protocol/PGD. This should be recorded in the patients notes

- When inflammation settles the tympanic membrane should be examined for middle ear disease

- Review if unsure of findings

- **Always** document, date, time and sign findings, treatment and advice given

AURAL CARE

- Patients should be warned not to let water into their ears and not to use anything to scratch their ears (cotton buds) Review Patient in 2 weeks

- If the condition resolved, give the patient an open appointment .

- If condition is still current, aural suction, review patient education, change medication if more than one sensitivity was given on swab report. Review as required for severity of condition, for chronic otitis externa this may be on a monthly basis. Each patient to be assessed individually.

Points to remember

- a patient may develop an allergy to ear drops
- regular use of ear drops may precipitate a fungal infection
- patient to use the full course of medication
- chronic Infection can be bacterial or fungal
- If unsure or condition fails to improve - refer
- record all findings and treatment given, match sticks

For uncomplicated AOE there appears to be no significant difference in outcomes when comparing different topical antimicrobial drops. If a perforation can be seen or one is unable to visualise the tympanic membrane it is best to use non-ototoxic drops such as quinolone topical drops as a first line treatmet. Non-ototoxic 0.3% ciprofloxacin eye drops can be used in the ear very effectively, however this is an unlicensed use in the UK and may require the addition of separate steroid drops. Aminoglycoside drops are an effective treatment for the severe discharging ear, although there is concern about ototoxicity the ENTUK consensus guidelines state they can be used in the presence of a perforation for a maximum of two weeks. The use of combined steroid and antimicrobial drops is more effective than steroid drops alone and appears better at improving symptoms than antibiotic drops alone.

GUIDELINES FOR THE TREATMENT OF MASTOID CAVITIES

Types of mastoid operations

Cortical performed to treat acute mastoiditis, surgical removal of the mastoid air cells leaving the ear canal and middle ear structures intact. Ear appears normal on examination and should self clean.

Radical performed to control cholesteatoma, surgical removal of mastoid air cells, tympanic membrane, ossicles and middle ear mucosa, creating a single large cavity.

AURAL CARE

Modified Radical   performed to control less extensive disease, tympanic membrane and ossicular chain preserved if possible.

Combined Approach   endaural/postaural approach to remove Tympanoplasty cholesteatoma avoiding destruction of hearing, often used in younger patients, appearance similar to cortical mastoidectomy.

Radical and some modified radical and atticotomies are unable to self clean and require regular aural toilet. Cortical mastoidectomies and combined approach tympanoplasties require aural toilet and dewaxing if necessary. All crusts need to be removed because there may be active disease behind them. Surgery is performed to remove small attic cholesteatoma, ossicular chain is left intact, size and shape of cavity depends on extent of disease.

1. **Cleaning the mastoid cavity**

    - Position patient under the microscope
    - Examine EAC, including meatal floor, the attic and posterior areas
    - If cavity dry - review 6 - 12 months
    - If cavity active - clean with micro-suction
    - Pearly, smelly mass or crusts indicates recurrence of Cholesteatoma - **REFER**

- Granular - Trimovate ointment, review 1 month, if unresolved - **REFER**
- If cavity discharging - clear debris with micro-suction. Otomise for 2 weeks, review 1 month, if unresolved - **REFER**

2. **Referral**

Recurrence of cholesteatoma
Chronically discharging cavity

GUIDELINES FOR THE TREATMENT OF FURUNCLE

A furuncle is a staphylococcal infection of the hair follicles found in the lateral part of the EAM. It presents with severe otalgia made worse by movement of the pinna and deafness. Examination is very difficult because of the pain. Most rupture spontaneously.

- Take a swab for culture and sensitivity

- Clean ear gently, as this is a very painful condition

- Insert a Glycerine and Icthammol wick daily if possible, until inflammation is reduced (if not possible, change after 24 hours and then as clinics permit)

- **REFER** for systemic antibiotics and analgesia

- Explain to patient condition will get better, importance of compliance with treatment and advise to rest until pain subsides

GUIDELINES FOR REMOVAL OF FOREIGN BODIES

Most commonly found in children (beads, cotton wool buds etc). May be accompanied by discharge, bleeding, deafness and/or pain. Co-operation and a good light source are necessary. Usually a child will allow only one attempt at removal which, if unsuccessful, will require a general anaesthetic. Therefore, if you think you will be unable to remove the object easily refer to the doctor. If inserted deeply into the EAC a perforation of the tympanic membrane can result. Objects such as peas, peanuts and vegetable matter will swell if liquid is put into the ear making removal difficult.

An object near the tympanic membrane is usually removed under general anaesthetic

1. Beads, stones and plastic objects

Position patient under microscope
   Assess position in EAM
   ***REFER** if unsure*
   Attempt removal with blunt hook or suction
   Assess tympanic membrane: discharge if intact – **REFER** if perforation
   Removal unsuccessful - **REFER**

2. Soft objects

   Position patient under microscope
   Assess position of object in EAM
   REFER if unsure
   Attempt removal with grasping forceps/suction
   Assess tympanic membrane, discharge if intact, **REFER** if perforation
   Removal unsuccessful, **REFER**

2. Insects

   Position patient under microscope
   Assess position and status of insect in EAC   - ***REFER* if unsure**
   If insect is alive instil olive oil, alcohol or spirit to drown it
   Attempt removal with suction or grasping forceps

AURAL CARE

Assess tympanic membrane, Discharge if intact , **REFER** if perforation
Removal unsuccessful - **REFER**

REFERRAL

Failed attempt at removal
Uncooperative child
Suspected trauma to tympanic membrane
Risk of damaging tympanic membrane during removal

GUIDELINES FOR THE MANUAL REMOVAL OF WAX

WAX

Ear Wax is a normal bodily secretion, it emerges from the external ear canal spontaneously, the skin from the lateral surface of the tympanic membrane is migratory travelling outwards from the ear drum and along the ear canal. Wax provides a protective film, therefore should only be removed if causing deafness, pain or it blocks the view of the tympanic membrane. Factors that prevent the normal extrusion of wax from the ear canal are wearing a hearing aid and patients attempting to clean their own ears with cotton buds. The wax is pushed deeper into the canal and compacted. Further attempts at removal can cause trauma and secondary otitis externa. Wax removal has been shown to improve hearing in-patients with impacted wax.

Soft wax should be removed by aural suction - care must be taken not to traumatise the meatal wall.

- If the wax is too hard to remove softening agents are the first line of management. Trying to remove hard wax can tear the meatal skin allowing a portal of entry for infection.

- Sodium bicarbonate eardrops for 5 days, 3-4 drops to the affected ear twice daily. If the patient has a perforation to tympanic membrane advise use of olive oil. Instructions as how to administer drops to be given to the patient.

- Review patients in 2 weeks. Examine ear to see if wax softened

- When wax is removed check the tympanic membrane, examine the attic area.

- If any cholesteatoma, retraction pockets or perforations, document and **refer** to doctor if these are new findings

- Document all observations, treatments (including rationale), information given to patient

- With patients with chronic wax problem, advise them to use olive oil on a prn????? basis to keep wax softer

- Arrange follow-up appointment or review

- Send letter outlining changes to treatment to GP

PROTOCOL FOR THE ADMINISTRATION OF AURAL MEDICATIONS

Medications for use by nurses in the Aural Dressing Clinic

Consider requesting the prescription of:

Otomize
Otitis externa
Chronic otitis externa Chronic itching

Locorteh Vioform
Dry/flaky ears or fungal infection

Sofradex
To clear out debris

Gentisone HC
Otitis externa

Ciprofloxacin
Otitis externa

Consider the application (via a 2ml ear syringe, gauze wick or popes wick) of creams and ointments –

Trimovate
Granulations present
Chronically discharging mastoid cavities
Otitis externa

Beclamethosone
Eczematous otitis externa
Suspicion of allergic reaction

Beclamethasone and Neomycin
Otitis externaInfected Mastoid cavities

AURAL CARE

Beclamethosone and Clioquinol
Otitis Externa
Infected mastoid cavities

Ichthalmol and Glycerine
Furunculosis

Clotrimazole
Fungal Infections

The decision on which preparation to use depends on the severity of the Otitis Externa and the patient's manual dexterity.

- Care should be taken with antibiotic ear preparations because antibiotics can cause allergic skin reactions. They may also cause growth of secondary infections such as fungi and worsen the condition.
- To instil drops, the head needs to be held with the ear uppermost and it is often easier for somebody else to put in the drops.
- Sprays are often easier for the patients to use themselves, and do not need specific positioning of the head. They do however need the ear canal to be fairly open.

Records must be kept of any patients experiencing adverse reactions and regular audit carried out.

Non-response to treatment is often due to inadequate cleaning of the ear canal.

Formal ENT-UK guidance for the use of aminoglycoside containing ear drops in the presence of a perforation As published in Clinical Otolaryngology;

AURAL CARE

Recommendation 1.
The following items have to be adopted (as formal ENT-UK guidance when treating a patient with a discharging ear, in whom there is a perforation or patent grommet. **If a topical aminoglycoside is used, this should only be in the presence of obvious infection. Topical aminoglycosides should be used for no longer than 2 weeks.** The justification for using topical aminoglycosides should be explained to the patient. Baseline audiometry should be performed, if possible or practical, before treatment with topical aminoglycosides.

Recommendation 2.
ENT-UK should seek expert advice on the use of ototopical quinolones, specifically on the advisability of their un-licensed use for patients with a discharging ear, in whom there is a perforation or patent grommet What are the potential adverse *effects* in terms of emergence of bacterial resistance?

Keypoints
- There seems to be little evidence linking vertigo or hearing loss to the short-term use of aminoglycoside-containing drops in discharging ears, in the presence of a grommet or perforation.

- The 'evidence' that does exist is of poor quality, consisting of data from a number of case reports and small case series.

- Prospective studies into the ototoxic effects of aminoglycoside ear drops either support their use but lack power to statistically confirm this, or are performed in conditions that are not representative of normal clinical conditions.

- Guidelines produced outside the UK recommend the use of quinolone-containing drops that are not licensed in this country.

- Although it is possible for individual doctors to use such drops 'off licence', it is appropriate that ENT-UK should issue guidance on the continued use of aminoglycoside-containing drops.

- Mindful of the need to produce clinical guidelines based on the best available evidence, the Clinical Audit and Practice Advisory Group of the British Association of Otolaryngologists – Head and Neck Surgeons (ENT-UK) has produced recommendations based on the views of an expert consensus panel.

9 PROTOCOLS

EXAMPLE PROTOCOL FOR AURAL MICRO-SUCTION

1) The Aural Dressing Clinic is staffed by a first level nurse who has completed a documented period of training under the supervision of an ENT surgeon and/or aural care nurse practitioner of not less than six months.

2) Clinics take place in the ENT Out-Patient department.

3) Case records are to be obtained, before treatment, for the assessment of previous dressing clinic treatments and recording of any new treatments given.

4) All new patient referral letters are seen by a doctor and marked 'dressing clinic'; the aural care nurse practitioner will assess priority for treatment, liaise with appointment staff and book patients accordingly.

5) All new patients will have an assessment record completed by the nurse practitioner on the patient's initial visit, documenting past medical history, condition, symptoms and treatment.

6) Each follow-up appointment will be allocated 20 minutes for discussion, treatment and documentation.

7) Verbal consent to treatment by a nurse must be obtained before any treatment.

8) Written guidelines for aural micro-suction must be adhered to.

9) Aural medications need to be administered according to the agreed protocols. The nurse practitioner needs to have completed a period of instruction and be signed competent by the ward manager, pharmacy and the ENT consultant as able to administer/dispense aural medication.

10) GPs to be informed by letter of their patients' treatment and/or discharge from clinic.

11) Any patient refusing treatment, wishing to see a doctor or presenting with a condition beyond the nurse's remit, must be given an appointment to see the next available doctor.

SUGGESTED TRAINING PROGRAMME

The aim is to provide the nurse with the knowledge and practical skills to use micro-suction in a safe, effective way.

Supervision

This must be by the consultant in charge of the department or a nominated advanced nurse practitioner.

Outcomes

The nurse should be able to
1. Describe the anatomy of a normal ear;
2. Recognise abnormal anatomy;
3. Understand basic ear conditions ie: otitis externa, wax, polyps, cholesteatoma;
4. Perform safe micro-suction;
5. Understand the contraindications to micro suction;
6. Understand the potential risks and know when to refer for a second opinion.

Part 1

Theoretical sessions to provide:
- Anatomy and physiology;
- Clinical risk and accountability;
- Basic examination of ears;
- Ear diseases;
- Contra indications to micro-suction.

Part 2

Practical Sessions to provide:
- A period of observation of micro-suction;
- Supervised micro-suction when the trainee feels competent to perform this. An agreed minimum number of cases needs to be established: for experienced ENT nurses this may be as little as 10 cases, but for others usually 30 (see appendix);
- A record of all cases seen and treated must be kept by the trainee nurse.

Part 3

Assessment of competence after independent treatment of an agreed number of cases, to be checked by the Consultant/Aural Nurse Practitioner

SUGGESTED EQUIPMENT REQUIRED TO SET UP AN AURAL CARE CLINIC

ENT microscope with teaching arm attachment 250mm lens/camera attachment;

Adjustable hi/lo examination couch/chair/stool;

1 suction machine, bottle and lengths of flexible tuning;

Mayo trolley or dressing trolley;

Suitable clinic room.

Range of Instruments

Aural speculums (oblique ended): set of five in varying sizes: No 3, No 4, No 5;

Zoellner suction tubes;

St Bart's model blunt wax hook;

Jobson Horne probes 5'/,";

Tilley aural dressing forceps;

Hartmann's aural forceps, crocodile, serrated edges, 2 sizes;

Storage facilities for instruments .

10 CASE STUDIES

CASE STUDY 1

A 25 year old man complains of acute right ear pain. He also noticed a watery discharge from the ear. He has recently returned from holiday abroad.

Symptoms
Pronounced ear pain, decreased hearing in the right ear and a thin watery discharge are present. Onset of symptoms occurred 5 days ago and they have been progressively worsening.

Relevant patient history
No history of allergies or acute otitis media. He has no OE history, but admitted to swimming daily whilst on holiday.

Physical findings
The patient exhibits guarding of the right ear and complains of tenderness when the tragus is manipulated during the examination. The ear canal appears severely inflamed, occluding the lumen of the canal. Little erythema is present. Swelling makes visualization of the tympanic membrane impossible.

Diagnosis
Diffuse acute bacterial OE.

Treatment
1. Gently clean the discharge from the ear canal and take a swab for culture and sensitivity;
2. Insert Trimovate wick;
3. Advise on analgesic;
4. Return in 24 hours and then provide antibiotic steroid drops eg Neomycin plus Betnesol or, when they become available in the UK, a Fluroquinolone and steroid combination.

It may be beneficial to insert a wick to ensure delivery of medication because of the degree of inflammation in this patient's ear canal.

Discussion
Use of the Aminoglycoside or Fluoroquinolones provides excellent coverage of the pathogens most frequently associated with OE. Unlike the Aminoglycoside-containing preparations, the Fluoroquinolones are not associated with any ototoxicity. The steroid component offers an additional benefit because it helps relieve inflammation and provides quicker resolution of pain.

Follow up
Advise the patient on the proper administration of the medication and emphasise the importance of finishing the course of therapy even if the symptoms resolve. Instruct the patient to return again if the condition does not improve or if it worsens.

CASE STUDY 2

A 69 year old woman complains of unresolved bacterial OE involving the left ear. Despite a 10 day course of therapy with Ear Calm (Hydrocortisone and Ascetic Acid Otic solution) the infection has not resolved.

Symptoms
Intense pain in the left ear, some loss of hearing, continued discharge.

Relevant patient history
In addition to the OE, the patient has a history of diabetes mellitus.

Physical findings
Examination of the ear reveals inflammation of the canal and some erythema.

Diagnosis
A diagnosis of *malignant OE* is made on the basis of the clinical findings and confirmed by a bone scan.

Treatment
Therapy is immediately instituted with a systemic antibacterial agent such as Ciprofloxacin with topical aminoglycoside antibiotic treatment.

Discussion

Several years ago the mortality associated with malignant OE was as high as 80%. Today, with the development of improved treatment modalities, the mortality has decreased to 3-4% . Combination oral and topical treatment is necessary to halt the progression of the infection. It is prudent to treat any diabetic patient with acute OE with a combination of topical and systemic antibiotic agents. If the patient appears toxic or has a cranial nerve palsy, then initial therapy with intravenous antibiotics in addition to topical agents should be employed.

CASE STUDY 3

A 14 year old girl returns to the clinic with itching and discharge of the left ear. She complains of having a "blocked up" ear.

Physical findings
Examination of the left ear reveals a thin, watery discharge and inflammation of the EAC. Hearing reduction is noted.

Relevant Patient History
The patient, a swimmer on the local school team, has a history of recurrent OE. Three days ago she had been diagnosed with acute OE and was prescribed Sofradex, Soframycin, Polymyxin B and Dexamethasone.

Diagnosis
Acute OE but possibly a topical reaction to Soframycin

Treatment

Immediately discontinue use of aminoglycosides, prescribe analgesia for pain relief. Use steroid cream wick (eg. Betnovate) if the condition is severe, and review after 2 days to assess improvement.

Discussion

Amino glycoside reactions are common (up to 1/3 of patients are affected) and can range from mild to severe. Patients will be advised to discontinue use of this agent. Additional medication will be prescribed (eg Fluoroquinolones, analgesics), and follow-up visits to the doctor are warranted .

Follow up

The patient is shown the proper administration techniques and is instructed to take the medication as prescribed. She is also told to call if the condition does not improve. If dermatitis or eczema are present at this time, then the patient should be treated with 2% Hydrocortisone cream. The cream should be used twice a day until the itching and flaking resolve and then twice a week for prophylaxis, as this agent may reduce the likelihood of recurrent OE. Most importantly she should use fitted ear plugs held in by a bathing cap when swimming or change her sport.

11 REFERENCES

Abelardo E, Pope L, Rajkumar K, Greenwood R, Nunez DA. A double-blind randomised clinical trial of the treatment of otitis externa using topical steroid alone versus topical steroid-antibiotic therapy.
Eur Arch Otorhinolaryngol. 2009;266(1):41-45.

Bapat U, Nia J, Bance M Severe audiovestibular loss following ear syringing for wax removal.
J Laryngol Otol. 2001 May;115(5):410-1

Bhattacharyya N, Kepnes LJ. Initial impact of the acute otitis externa clinical practice guideline on clinical care. Otolaryngol Head Neck Surg. 2011;145(3):414-417.

Browning GG Ear wax.
BMJ Clin Evid. 2008 Jan 25;2008

Burton MJ, Doree C Ear drops for the removal of ear wax
Cochrane Database Syst Rev. 2009 Jan 21;(1)

Clegg AJ, Loveman E, Gospodarevskaya E, Harris P, Bird A, Bryant J, Scott DA, Davidson P, Little P, Coppin R. The safety and effectiveness of different methods of earwax removal: a systematic review and economic evaluation.
Health Technol Assess. 2010 Jun;14(28):1-192

Coppin R, Wicke D, Little P Managing earwax in primary care: efficacy of self-treatment using a bulb syringe

Br J Gen Pract. 2008 Jan;58(546):44-9

Eekhof JA, de Bock GH, Le Cessie S, Springer MP A quasi-randomised controlled trial of water as a quick softening agent of persistent earwax in general practice.
Br J Gen Pract. 2001 Aug;51(469):635-7.

Hawke M Update on cerumen and ceruminolytics.
Ear Nose Throat J. 2002 Aug;81(8 Suppl 1):23-4.

Kaushik V, Malik T, Saeed SR. Interventions for acute otitis externa.
Cochrane Database Syst Rev. 2010(1):CD004740.

Kumar S, Kumar M, Lesser T, Banhegyi G. Foreign bodies in the ear: a simple technique for removal analysed in vitro
Emerg Med J. 2005 Apr;22(4):266-8

Macfadyen CA, Acuin JM, Gamble C. Systemic antibiotics versus topical treatments for chronically discharging ears with underlying eardrum perforations.
Cochrane Database Syst Rev. 2006(1)

Memel D, Langley C, Watkins C, Laue B, Birchall M, Bachmann M. Effectiveness of ear syringing in general practice: a randomised controlled trial and patients' experiences.
Br J Gen Pract. 2002 Nov;52(484):906-11

National Institute for Health and Care Excellence, Clinical Knowledge Summaries, Otitis Externa. Revised July 2015

Pabla L, Jindal M, Latif K. The management of otitis externa in UK general practice.
Eur Arch Otorhinolaryngol. 2012;269(3):753-756.

Phillips JS, Yung MW, Burton MJ, Swan IR. Evidence review and ENT-UK consensus report for the use of aminoglycoside-containing ear drops in the presence of an open middle ear.
Clin Otolaryngol. 2007;32(5):330-336.

Roland PS, Stewart MG, Hannley M, Friedman R, Manolidis S, Matz G et al. Consensus panel on role of potentially ototoxic antibiotics for topical middle ear use: Introduction, methodology, and recommendations.
Otolaryngol Head Neck Surg. 2004;130(3 Suppl):S51-56.

Rosenfeld RM, Singer M, Wasserman JM, Stinnett SS. Systematic review of topical antimicrobial therapy for acute otitis externa.
Otolaryngol Head Neck Surg. 2006;134(4 Suppl):S24-48.

Rosenfeld RM, Schwartz SR, Cannon CR, Roland PS, Simon GR, Kumar KA et al. Clinical practice guideline: acute otitis externa.
Otolaryngol Head Neck Surg. 2014;150(1 Suppl):S1-S24.

Rowlands S, Devalia H, Smith C, Hubbard R, Dean A. Otitis externa in UK general practice: a survey using the UK General Practice Research Database.
Br J Gen Pract. 2001;51(468):533-538.

Sharp JF, Wilson JA, Ross L, Barr-Hamilton RM Ear wax removal: a survey of current practice.
BMJ. 1990 Dec 1;301(6763):1251-3.

Thomas AM1, Poojary B, Badaridatta HC Facial nerve palsy as a complication of ear syringing.
J Laryngol Otol. 2012 Jul;126(7):714-6.

Tshifularo M, Masotja MS Ruptured internal carotid artery aneurysm presenting with bloody otorrhoea and epistaxis as a result of ear syringing
S Afr J Surg. 2008 Nov;46(4):136

Woollons A, Price ML Roaccutane and wax epilation: a cautionary tale.
Br J Dermatol. 1997 Nov;137(5):839-40.

Wright T Ear wax.
BMJ Clin Evid. 2015 Mar 4;2015. pii: 0504.
further reading
KEY TOPICS IN OTOLARYNGOLOGY AND HEAD AND NECK SURGERY (DATE) Eds. Rowland N., and McCray D Butterworths.

TABLE FOR TRAINING

- Conditions Observed and treated should cover the spectrum of outer and middle ear diseases covered in the guide.

- There is no need to complete the observed conditions before moving onto the directly supervised.

- The observed can be done at the same time as the directly supervised but not on the same ear.

- Likewise the training by direct supervision can overlap with the training by review of patient after the procedure is carried out.

- Nurse Trainee Reflection is one of the most important parts of the process. What did I do? Why did I do it? Could I have done it better? What did I learn about the condition? What did I learn about my skills? Did I document well? Can I treat the same problem/patient well again?

- Thirty of each type of condition, observed, supervised and reviewed after doing, are required for new trainees.

\multicolumn{4}{c	}{**OBSERVE THE CONDITION BEING TREATED**}
DATE	CONDITION TREATED	SUPERVISOR SIGNATURE	REFLECTION AND LEARNING POINTS

AURAL CARE

SIGNED OFF BY SUPERVISOR   DATE

SUPERVISED/WATCHED BY SUPERVISOR				
DATE	CONDITION TREATED	SUPERVISOR SIGNATURE	REFLECTION AND LEARNING POINTS	

AURAL CARE

SIGNED OFF BY SUPERVISOR   DATE

DONE BY TRAINEE AND REVIEWED BY SUPERVISOR				
DATE	CONDITION TREATED	SUPERVISOR SIGNATURE	REFLECTION AND LEARNING POINTS

AURAL CARE

SIGNED OFF BY SUPERVISOR   DATE

Printed in Great Britain
by Amazon